Illustrated Pocket Guide to

Clinical
Medicine

Illustrated Pocket Guide to

Clinical
Medicine

Charles D Forbes DSc MD FRCP FRSE
Professor of Medicine
Ninewells Hospital and Medical School
Dundee
Scotland

William F Jackson MA MB BChir MRCP
Medical Writer
Formely Honorary Consultant
Department of Medicine
Guy's Hospital
London
England

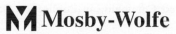
Mosby-Wolfe

London Baltimore Barcelona Bogotá Boston Buenos Aires Caracas Carlsbad, CA Chicago Madrid Mexico City Milan
New York Philadelphia St Louis Seoul Singapore Sydney Taipei Tokyo Toronto Wiesbaden

Published in 1997 by Mosby-Wolfe, an imprint of Times Mirror
International Publishers Limited

Printed by Grafos, Arte sobre papel, Barcelona, Spain

ISBN 0 7234 2951 0

For full details of all Times Mirror International Publishers Limited
titles, please write to Times Mirror International Publishers
Limited, Lynton House, 7–12 Tavistock Square, London WC1H
9LB, England.

A CIP catalogue record for this book is available from the British
Library.

Library of Congress Cataloging-in-Publication Data applied for.

PREFACE

This *Illustrated Pocket Guide* contains 525 pictures selected from the total of over 1700 pictures that appear in the second edition of Forbes & Jackson's *Color Atlas and Text of Clinical Medicine*. We have prepared this book in response to specific requests from two groups of potential readers.

Firstly, we have been asked for a pocket version of our larger book which can be used for instant reference or revision purposes in any situation—especially by students and junior physicians on the wards, and by candidates preparing for clinical and picture-test examinations at undergraduate and postgraduate level.

Secondly, we have been asked for a book of clinical pictures, which can be used as a supplement to large, essentially unillustrated textbooks of medicine, and to the many texts used by paramedics, nurses, physiotherapists and others in the professions allied to medicine. Although our larger book has been much used by these groups, it is clear that many readers would value a smaller, pocket-sized book containing pictures without additional text.

In making our selection of pictures for the *Illustrated Pocket Guide*, we have aimed to meet the needs of both these groups of readers. We have tried to select the pictures which are of most widespread clinical relevance, while still maintaining a comprehensive coverage of the core of clinical medicine, and following the chapter structure of the larger book. We have modified many of the picture legends for this 'stand alone' use, and as far as possible they contain key points about all the conditions illustrated. For further information, the reader should refer to Forbes & Jackson's *Color Atlas and Text of Clinical Medicine* or to other medical texts.

As in the larger book, we are grateful to those who have allowed us to use their pictures. They are listed overleaf. In all cases, however, responsibility for picture selection, relevance and description rests with us. Our preparation of this book over a short period, at the same time as we were working on the final stages of the second edition of the larger book and meeting many other commitments has stretched the tolerance of our wives, Janette Forbes and Barbara Jackson, to its limit. As always, we are grateful to them for their continued support.

Charles Forbes, Dundee
William Jackson, Oxford

ACKNOWLEDGEMENTS

We gratefully acknowledge the generosity of the many colleagues and institutions listed below, who lent us single, or in a few cases, multiple pictures.

CDF and WFJ

G Allan, Glasgow, UK
M C Allison, Newport, UK
J Anderson, Dundee, UK
M Baraitser, London, UK
J F Belch, Dundee, UK
M Berger, Sydney, Australia
A B Bridges, Stirling, UK
J C Brocklehurst, Manchester, UK
R Cerio, London, UK
G S J Chessell, Aberdeen, UK
G M Cochrane, London, UK
W B Conolly, Sydney, Australia
A Cuschieri, Dundee, UK
D Davidson, Dundee, UK
J Dequeker, Leuven, Belgium
V Dubowitz, London, UK
K Duguid, Aberdeen, UK
D L Easty, Bristol, UK
C F Farthing, Los Angeles, USA
N J R George, Manchester, UK
H M Gilles, Liverpool, UK
H W Gray, Glasgow, UK
J Hanslip, Dundee, UK
CA Hart, Liverpool, UK
L K Jackson, Swindon, UK
M J Jamieson, Aberdeen, UK
R Johnston, Dundee, UK
M Jones, Dundee, UK
R T Jung, Dundee, UK
A Kamal, Lincoln, UK
N Kennedy, Dundee, UK
The estate of the late L Kessel, London, UK
E E Kritzinger, Birmingham, UK
R E Latchaw, Minneapolis, USA
R W Lloyd-Davies, London, UK
C Lockie, Stratford-upon-Avon, UK

J G Lowe, Dundee, UK
C J McEwan, Dundee, UK
D S McLaren, London, UK
W McNab, Dundee, UK
G P McNeill, Dundee, UK
R McTier, Glasgow, UK
K L G Mills, Aberdeen, UK
S Morley, Dundee, UK
R Morton, Chelmsford, UK
A Muir, Dundee, UK
R Newton, Dundee, UK
M Nimmo, Dundee, UK
C O'Callaghan, Leicester, UK
G Page, Aberdeen, UK
C R Pennington, Dundee, UK
W Peters, London, UK
J C Petrie, Aberdeen, UK
M J Pippard, Dundee, UK
S D Pringle, Dundee, UK
N K Ragge, London, UK
P J Rees, London, UK
M B Rubens, London, UK
M A Sambrook, Manchester, UK
A Seaton, Dundee, UK
K F R Schiller, Oxford, UK
M F Shiu, Coventry, UK
D J Sinclair, Edinburgh, UK
R C D Staughton, London, UK
P Sweny, London, UK
C Thompson, Glasgow, UK
H M A Towler, Aberdeen, UK
M Turner–Warwick, London, UK
W R Tyldesley, Liverpool, UK
S R Underwood, London, UK
United Medical and Dental Schools, Guy's Campus, London, UK (by courtesy of the Dean)

D Veale, Leeds, UK
W F Walker, Dundee, UK
S Walton, Aberdeen, UK
D A Warrell, Oxford, UK
Wellcome Institute Library, London,
UK
G Williams, Manchester, UK
J H Winter, Dundee, UK
A Wisdom, London, UK
V Wright, Leeds, UK

CONTENTS

1 **HIV-related rash** in a homosexual man. In addition to this rash, the patient presented with fever, sore throat and headache. Seroconversion was noted 5 weeks later.

2 **Painless lymph node enlargement in HIV infection** may develop at the time of seroconversion but usually resolves. Progressive lymph node enlargement may occur at a later stage.

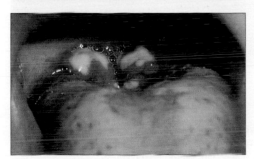

3 **Gross tonsillar enlargement** in an HIV-infected patient (CDC Group III).

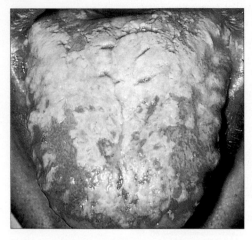

4 Extensive oral infection with *Candida albicans* in a patient with HIV infection. Note the gross changes in the tongue and the angular cheilitis.

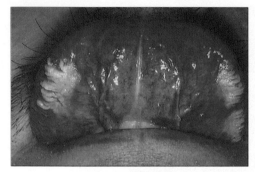

5 Hairy leukoplakia in a patient with HIV infection (CDC Group IV C$_2$). Note the appearance of a ribbed whiteness along the sides of the tongue.

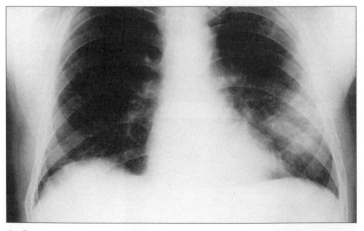

6 *Pneumocystis* **pneumonia** is the most common life-threatening opportunistic infection in patients with AIDS. In this patient there is consolidation in the left lower zone, but the changes may be more widespread.

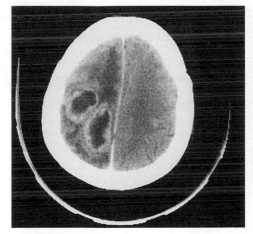

7 Cerebral abscesses in the right occipital region on a contrast-enhanced CT scan. In patients with HIV infection, the most common cause of cerebral abscess is *Toxoplasma gondii*, and the abscesses are often multiple.

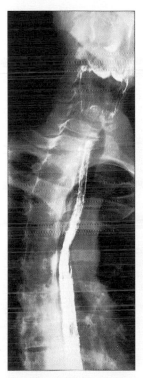

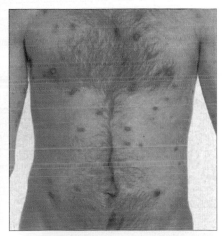

8 Candidiasis of the oesophagus in a patient with AIDS, demonstrated by barium swallow. Note the mottled appearance, which results from multiple plaques of candidiasis on the oesophageal mucosa.

9 Kaposi's sarcoma is a common complication in patients with AIDS, especially in those who contracted the disease by sexual transmission. Note the generalized lesions, many of which show peripheral bruising.

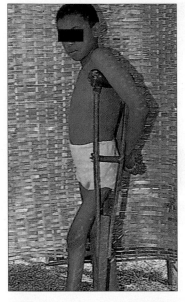

10 Paralysis of the left leg as a result of poliomyelitis. The disease is still a major problem in developing countries.

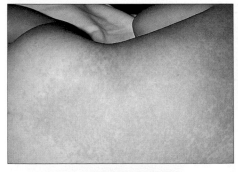

11 Rubella rash on the trunk. On the first day, the rash consists of discrete, delicate pink macules. These may coalesce on the second day, as here. The rash may be missed altogether when the lesions are sparse.

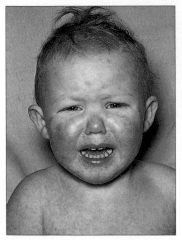

12 Measles. This miserable child has a characteristic appearance, with a fine, light red maculopapular rash on the face and trunk.

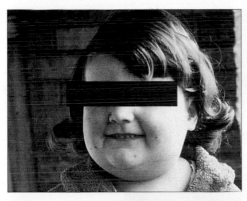

13 Mumps. There is marked bilateral enlargement of the parotid glands, which are usually tender, associated with generalized facial oedema.

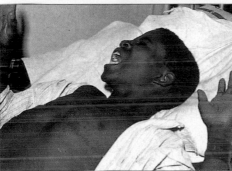

14 'Furious rabies' in a 14-year-old Nigerian boy. Inspiratory spasms occur spontaneously or are induced by attempts to swallow.

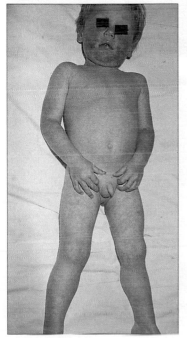

15 Erythema infectiosum. The erythematous rash appeared 24 hours after the onset of a mild fever and sore throat. Note the 'slapped cheek' appearance of the face.

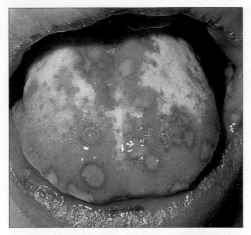

16 Severe herpetic gingivostomatitis. This young child was acutely ill with a high fever and had multiple vesicular lesions on the tongue, lips and buccal mucosa.

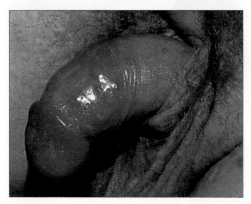

17 Primary genital herpes. Note the numerous lesions on the penis and the associated tissue reaction.

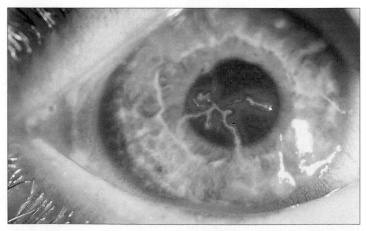

18 A primary herpetic dendritic ulcer, stained with fluorescein. Herpes simplex virus proliferates in the epithelial layer of the cornea. Urgent treatment with antiviral therapy is indicated.

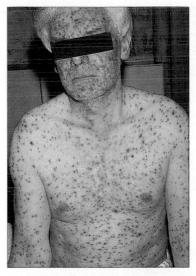

19 Chicken-pox in an adult patient. The lesions emerge in crops at irregular intervals, and this patient shows vesicles at different stages of development.

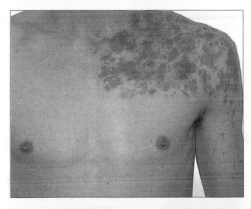

20 Herpes zoster (shingles) showing a characteristic 'band' distribution, here affecting left dermatomes C4 and C5.

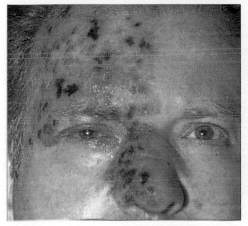

21 Ophthalmic herpes. The vesicular skin eruptions are in the distribution of the ophthalmic division of the fifth cranial nerve. Serious ophthalmic complications may occur.

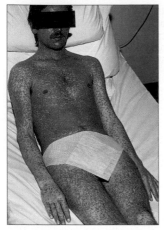

22 Rash in infectious mononucleosis may be the result of the infection itself or of the administration of ampicillin or related penicillin compounds.

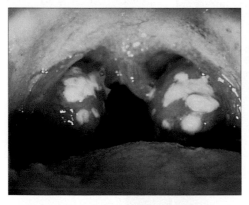

23 Infectious mononucleosis. In many patients there is tonsillitis, indistinguishable from that seen in acute streptococcal pharyngitis. Here there is pus in the tonsillar crypts, and some palatal petechiae are also seen.

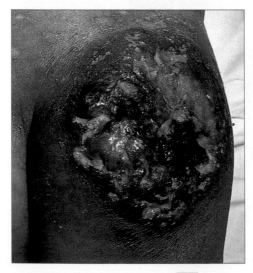

24 A massive staphylococcal carbuncle in a diabetic. The infection has caused tissue breakdown and multiple interconnected abscesses.

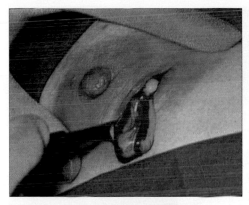

25 Drainage of a staphylococcal abscess. A large volume of pus was released when it was incised.

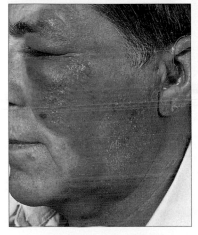

26 Erysipelas of the face results from infection with *Streptococcus pyogenes.* The entire face may become erythematous and oedematous.

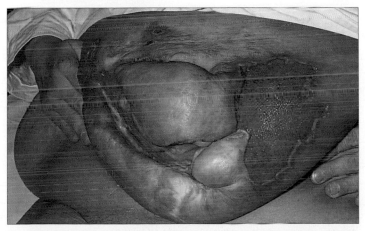

27 Necrotizing fascitis following surgical 'apronectomy' for extreme obesity. There is extensive cellulitis and erysipelas, and the subcutaneous infection was extensive and accompanied by gas formation and crepitus.

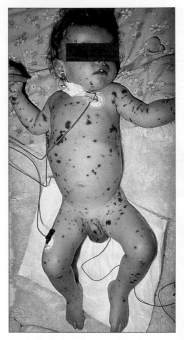

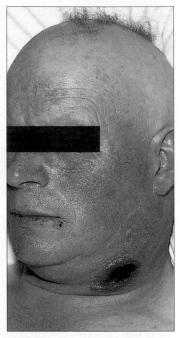

28 Fulminating meningococcal septicaemia is characterized by extensive purpuric lesions, a high fever, shock and evidence of disseminated intravascular coagulation.

29 Anthrax. A malignant pustule in a typical position on the neck. The patient was a porter who carried animal hides over his shoulders.

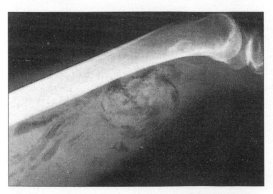

30 Gas gangrene in the soft tissues of the thigh after a penetrating injury. The combination of myonecrosis and gas results in swelling and impaired distal circulation.

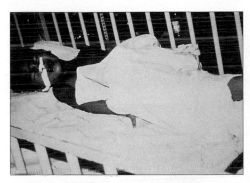

31 Tetanus. Tetanic spasms are painful, and the appearance of pain is accentuated by spasm of the facial muscles, giving a characteristic 'grin' (risus sardonicus).

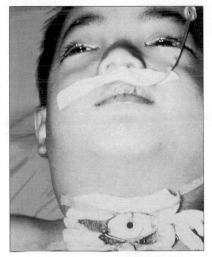

32 Diphtheria. Respiratory obstruction is a life-threatening complication and urgent tracheostomy may be essential. This child has a palatal palsy (hence the nasogastric tube), and a 'bull neck' (a characteristic appearance of cervical oedema).

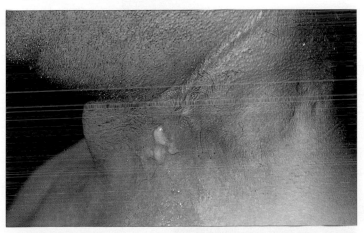

33 Cervical actinomycosis. The chronic nature of the condition is demonstrated by the signs of a previous sinus higher up in the neck, which has healed, and an actively discharging sinus below it.

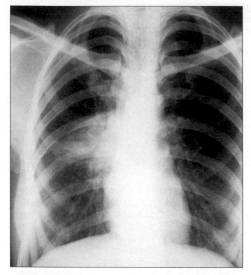

34 Primary tuberculosis. The primary focus is in the apical segment of the right lower lobe and there is also slight hilar enlargement.

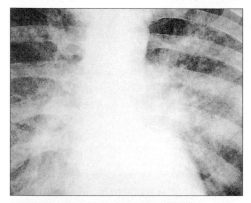

35 Miliary tuberculosis. Similar radiological appearances may be found in other forms of pneumonia, in sarcoidosis and in some occupational lung diseases.

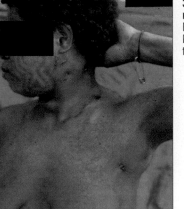

36 Enlarged tuberculous lymph nodes in the neck and axilla of a Fijian woman with widespread TB. Discharging sinuses are visible in the axilla and at the angle of the jaw.

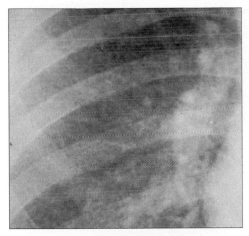

37 Hilar node enlargement is a common finding in tuberculosis, usually in association with pulmonary involvement.

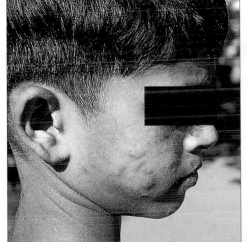

38 Lepromatous leprosy. There is infiltration and oedema of the cheek and thickening of the ear.

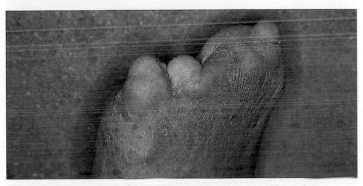

39 Neurotrophic atrophy in lepromatous leprosy eventually leads to erosion of the extremities.

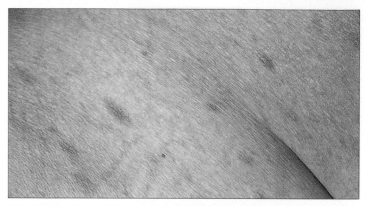

40 Typhoid fever. These typical rose spots are pinkish macules or maculopapules on the trunk, measuring 2–4 mm in diameter. The spots blanch on pressure.

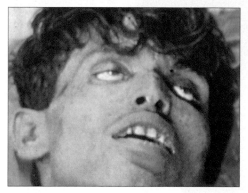

41 Cholera. Extreme dehydration has led to the typical appearance of deeply sunken cheeks and eyes. Rehydration can lead to complete recovery if started before the onset of renal failure.

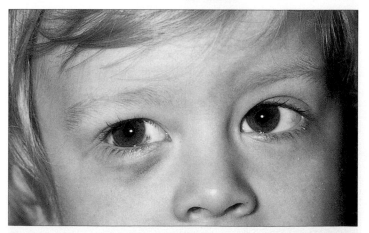

42 Pertussis. Subconjunctival haemorrhage occurs because the intrathoracic pressure rises sharply during violent paroxysms of coughing and leads to sudden surges in capillary pressure. Bleeding into the lower lid is a rarer complication.

**44 Allergic broncho-
pulmonary aspergillo-
sis,** showing widespread
changes of bronchiocta
sis, predominantly central
in distri-bution, with associated fibrotic scarring.

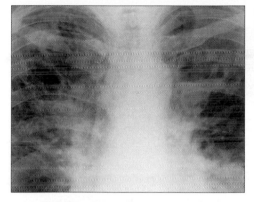

43 Lyme disease.
Erythema chronicum
migrans is the char-
acteristic rash. Note
the chronic indura-
tion, with a red mar-
gin and central clear-
ing.

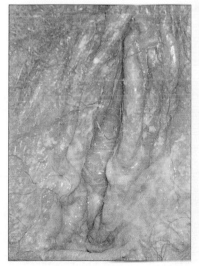

45 Candidiasis. Vaginal thrush is a
common problem in adult women
during or after antibiotic treatment,
in pregnancy and during oral contraceptive use. The curdy white discharge is characteristic.

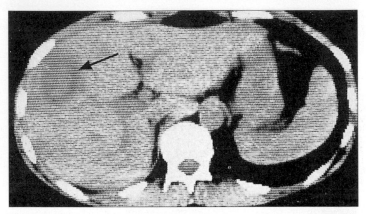

46 Amoebic liver abscess (arrowed) on CT scan in a British woman who had returned from vacation in Kenya 2 months earlier. She presented with right upper quadrant pain and fever.

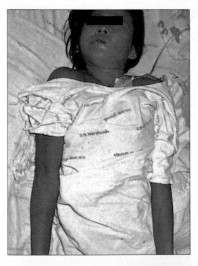

47 Cerebral malaria, with classic decerebrate rigidity in a Thai woman.

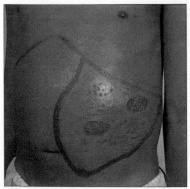

48 Chronic malaria may lead to the tropical splenomegaly syndrome (TSS). Note the outline of the massive spleen. The scars result from the local application of traditional healing techniques.

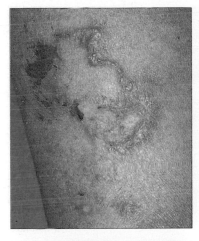

49 Cutaneous larva migrans, resulting from the migration of non-human hookworm larvae. The skin lesion was erythematous and itchy, and the patient had a marked eosinophilia.

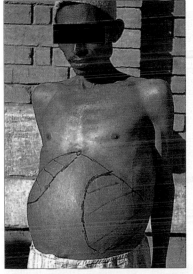

50 Schistosomiasis causing massive hepatosplenomegaly. The greatly enlarged spleen is accompanied by an enlarged irregularly fibrosed liver. The appearance is typical of infection with *S. mansoni.*

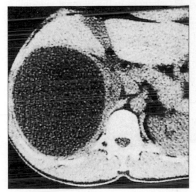

51 Massive hydatid cyst *(Echinococcus granulosus)* in the liver of a 14-year-old Kuwaiti boy, demonstrated by CT scanning.

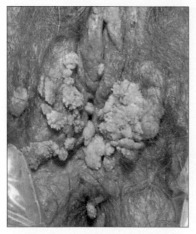

52 Florid labial, perineal and perianal warts. Genital warts vary greatly in appearance. They may be sessile, filiform or hyperplastic.

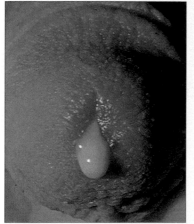

53 Gonorrhoea. The typical purulent urethral discharge can often be demonstrated during examination by 'milking' the urethra. The patient also has associated meatitis.

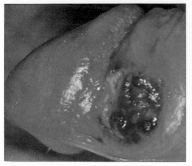

54 Syphilis – typical primary chancre in the coronal sulcus. A small red macule enlarges and develops through a papular stage, becoming eroded to form a typical round, painless ulcer. If untreated, the ulcer usually heals after 4–8 weeks.

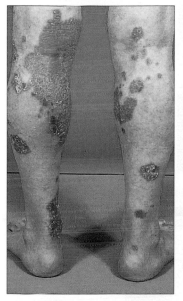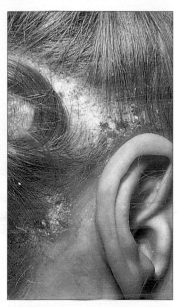

55 Psoriasis. Typical lesions on the legs. Further plaques were present on the extensor surfaces of the legs and arms.

56 Psoriasis of the scalp and hair margin. The patchy nature of scalp involvement helps to distinguish psoriasis from other conditions, such as dandruff and seborrhoeic dermatitis.

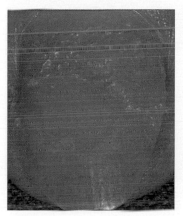

57 Psoriasis affecting the nail, causing pitting, onycholysis, discoloration and thickening.

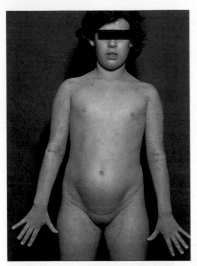

58 Flexural atopic dermatitis in the typical childhood distribution. As the lesions are itchy, they are usually scratched and lichenification may result. Even non-flexural skin is dry and may be itchy.

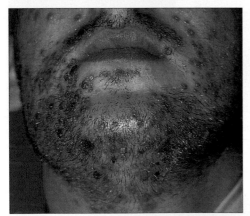

59 Secondary infection is common in eczema. This man has a herpes simplex infection (eczema herpeticum), which has prevented him from shaving.

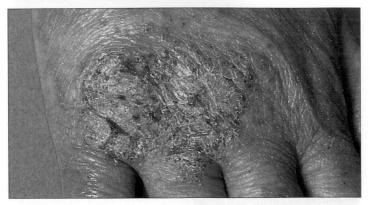

60 Discoid dermatitis. The condition often occurs in patients who have no previous history of atopic dermatitis. In this patient the lesions are 'weeping' serous fluid.

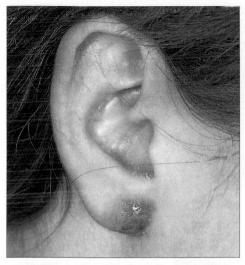

61 Contact dermatitis to nickel affects 10% of European women. Nickel is a common component of jewellery such as rings, necklaces and earrings.

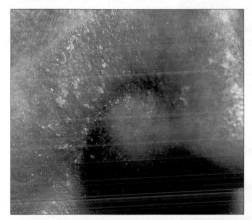

62 Florid seborrhoeic dermatitis showing typical red, scaly lesions. This is a common problem in HIV infection, but most patients with seborrhoeic dermatitis are not infected with HIV.

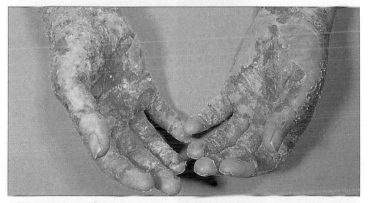

63 Irritant dermatitis on the hands of a 39-year-old man. It resulted from exposure to irritant chemicals at work.

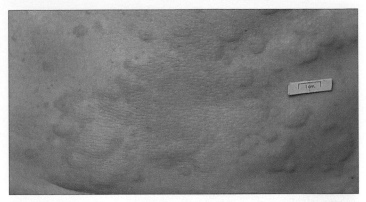

64 Urticaria in close-up, showing characteristic weals, surrounded by an erythematous flare.

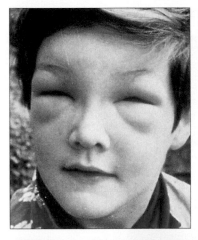

65 Severe angioedema in a 9-year-old boy after a bee sting. The patient required immediate treatment with adrenalin to overcome a generalized anaphylactic response.

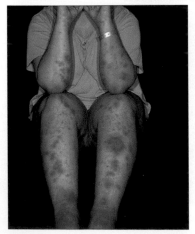

66 Erythema nodosum occurring in a classic distribution over the front of the legs and forearms. Further investigation revealed an underlying diagnosis of sarcoidosis.

67 Erythema multiforme usually starts with a symmetrical eruption of target-like lesions on the hands and feet. These may blister centrally and they spread proximally. The underlying cause was sulphonamide therapy.

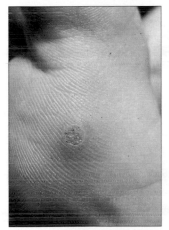

68 A plantar viral wart, popularly known as a 'verruca'. Single and multiple plantar warts are common, especially in school children.

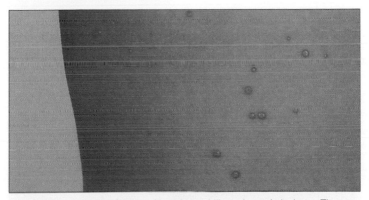

69 Molluscum contagiosum. Note the umbilicated, pearly lesions. The condition occurs in childhood and in otherwise normal adults, but it is particularly common in patients with HIV infection.

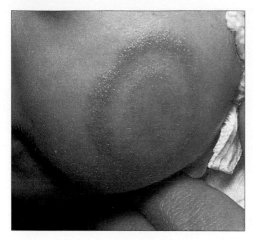

70 Tinea (ringworm). Note the scaly margins, which can be scraped and examined for fungal hyphae and spores. This florid case resulted from infection with *Micro-sporum canis.*

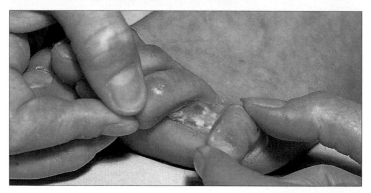

71 Tinea pedis ('athlete's foot') is a very common infection, especially in those who wear tight or poorly ventilated footwear.

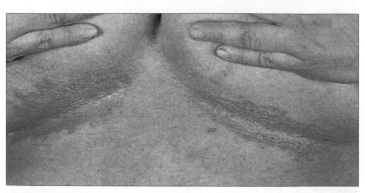

72 Candidiasis of the skin (intertriginous candidiasis) below both breasts in an obese diabetic.

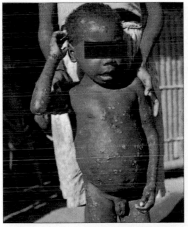

73   Scabies with secondary infected eczema in a boy from Papua.

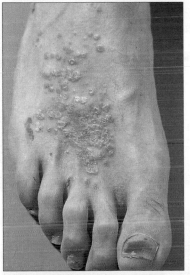

74 Lichen planus. The polygonal papules on the dorsum of the foot are typical of the chronic form of the disorder, and the lesions are commonly itchy.   Dystrophic nail changes are common in lichen planus.

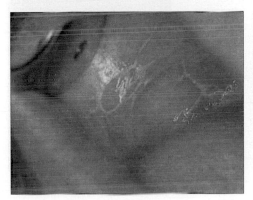

75 Oral lesions are relatively common in lichen planus. The classic appearance is of white reticulations on the buccal mucosa, as here, but the disease may also take an erosive form.

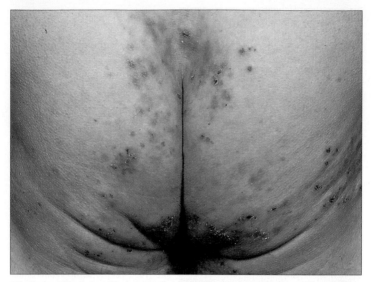

76 Dermatitis herpetiformis in the sacral and buttock areas. The vesicles have been ruptured by scratching, and are healing, leaving pigmented scars.

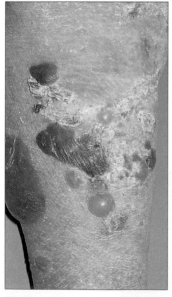

77 Pemphigoid. Some of the blisters have become haemorrhagic, as often occurs.

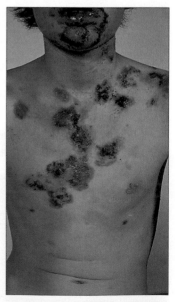

78 Pemphigus vulgaris. The blisters rupture easily, and are often associated with similar lesions on mucous membranes, especially in the mouth.

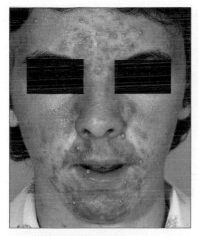

79 Acne vulgaris usually involves the face. This 17-year-old has many papular and pustular lesions at different stages of evolution, and the older lesions are healing with scarring.

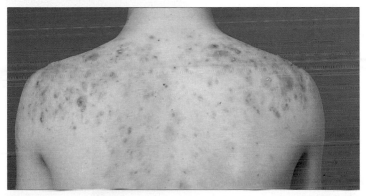

80 Acne vulgaris on the shoulders and back. Again, a wide range of lesions are seen, including some large pustules, and scarring is occurring on healing.

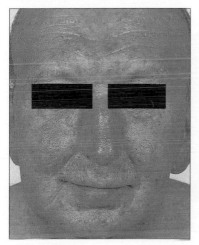

81 Acne rosacea. This patient shows typical papules and pustules, superimposed on a generally erythematous facial skin.

27

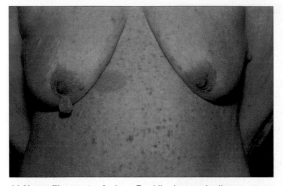

82 Neurofibromatosis (von Recklinghausen's disease, type 1). Note the subcutaneous nodular tumours arising in the sheaths of peripheral nerves, the pigmented pedunculated tumours on the skin surface and the brown (café-au-lait) patches.

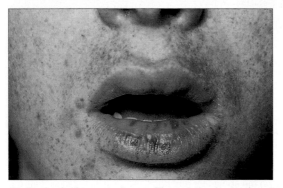

83 Peutz–Jeghers syndrome. Pigmentation is also found on the hard and soft palate, buccal mucosa and, occasionally, on the feet and hands. There is an association with multiple intestinal polyps.

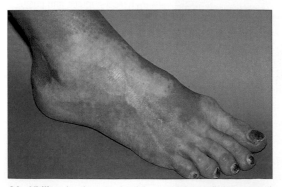

84 Vitiligo is characterized by multiple, well-demarcated areas of hypopigmentation that progressively enlarge. It is often associated with other autoimmune disorders.

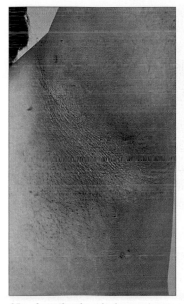

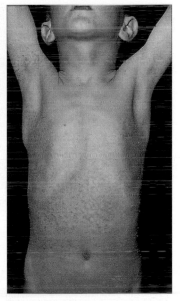

85 Acanthosis nigricans in an Asian patient. Patchy velvety brown hyperpigmentation and thickening of flexures develops. This is often a marker of underlying malignant disease, but it may occur in diabetes and other endocrine disorders or in isolation.

86 Ichthyosis vulgaris is a dominant condition that causes scaly skin from early childhood onwards. Its name reflects the resemblance of the skin to scaly fish skin.

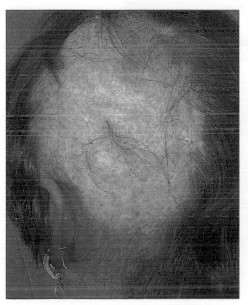

87 Severe alopecia areata in a 24-year-old woman. There are no features to suggest infection of the scalp.

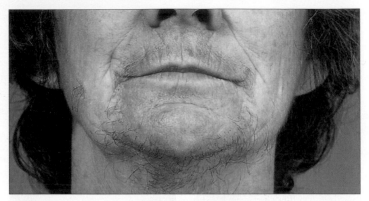

88 Hirsutism was the presenting symptom in this woman who was found to have an arrhenoblastoma.

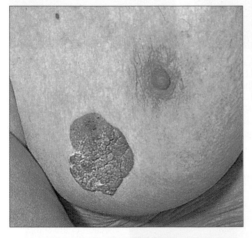

89 Seborrhoeic keratosis (seborrhoeic wart). These benign lesions are increasingly common with age, and they appear predominantly on unexposed Caucasian skin.

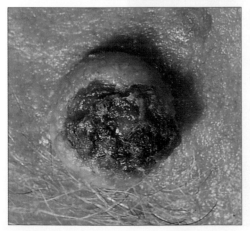

90 Keratoacanthoma on the neck. This ulcerating tumour, with a central keratin plug, grows rapidly but resolves spontaneously.

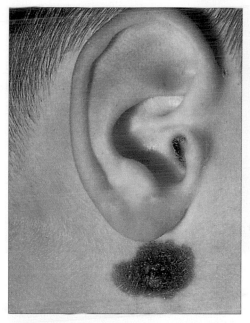

91 Benign melanocytic naevus (mole). This is benign, but if it were to change in shape, pigmentation or size, or if it were to bleed, biopsy would be necessary.

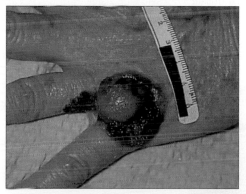

92 Malignant melanoma on the hand. The centre of the tumour is now amelanotic, but the local invasion remains pigmented and the patient had widespread secondary deposits.

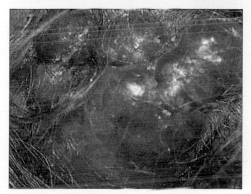

93 Skin secondaries, in this case in the scalp from a primary carcinoma of the bronchus. Such lesions are relatively uncommon.

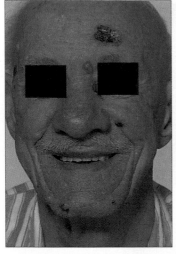

94 Multiple basal cell carcinomas.
The lesion on the bridge of the nose is typical of the common presentation as a slowly enlarging nodule. The other lesions demonstrate various stages of progression to rodent ulcers.

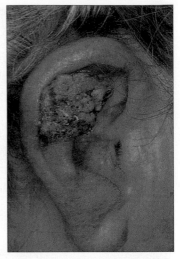

95 Squamous cell carcinoma begins as a small nodule, but slowly grows to produce the typical lesion seen here. The ulcer has thick edges and an irregular granular base; it usually produces a serous discharge.

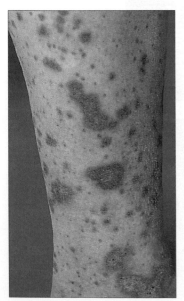

96 Leucocytoclastic vasculitis, with widespread, painful, palpable purpura on both legs. The lesions result from the deposition of immune complexes in the postcapillary venules.

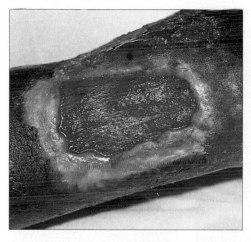

97 Pyoderma gangrenosum. There is a tender, superficial necrotic ulcer with a typical purple undermined edge. Pyoderma gangrenosum is suggestive of underlying systemic disease.

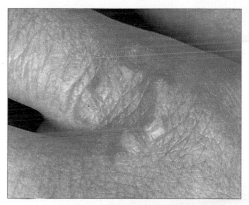

98 Granuloma annulare on the finger. Note the ring of flesh-coloured papules. This condition may occur in otherwise healthy individuals or in patients with diabetes.

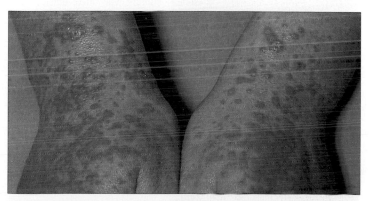

99 Polymorphic light eruption with typical itchy erythematous papules over the forearms and hands. The reaction most commonly appears within 24 hours of exposure to the sun.

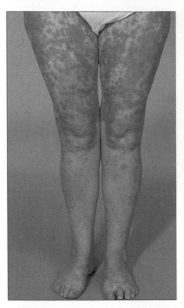

100 Drug rashes often present as a symmetrical erythematous maculopapular eruption. This patient had a history of previous penicillin rashes, which had not been taken into account when ampicillin was prescribed.

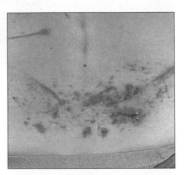

101 Phytophotodermatitis most commonly presents as irregular streaks of erythema and hyperpigmentation occurring on the light-exposed parts of the body. This gardener's skin had been exposed to giant hogweed.

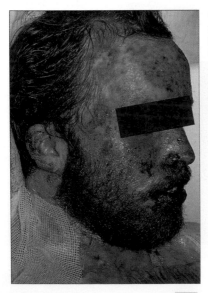

102 Stevens–Johnson syndrome is a widespread erythema multiforme with oral, genital and conjunctival involvement, and widespread skin lesions. It may occur as a drug reaction or following *Mycoplasma pneumoniae* infection.

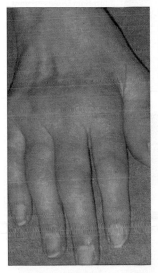

103   Rheumatoid arthritis. Note the swelling of the metacarpophalangeal and the proximal interphalangeal joints, subluxation with ulnar deformity, a fixed flexion deformity in the first metacarpophalangeal joint and disuse atrophy of the intrinsic muscles of the hands.

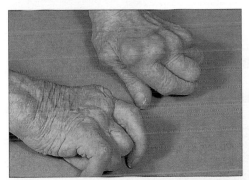

104   Chronic rheumatoid arthritis. The finger joints are not acutely inflamed, but there is polyarthritis with major residual deformity of the hand.

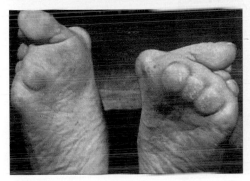

105 Rheumatoid arthritis in the feet. Gross destructive changes with multiple subluxations cause painful deformity that severely limits its mobility.

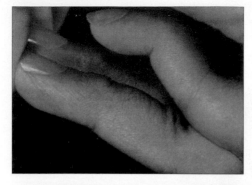

106 Swan-neck deformity is common in advanced rheumatoid arthritis. It results from disruption of the volar plate of the proximal interphalangeal joint, sometimes with associated rupture of the insertion of the flexor sublimis.

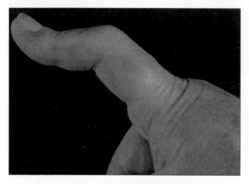

107 Boutonnière deformity. This common deformity in advanced rheumatoid arthritis results from the rupture of the central slip of the extensor tendon over the proximal interphalangeal joint. The lateral slips of the extensor tendon mechanism are displaced to the sides and maintain the deformity.

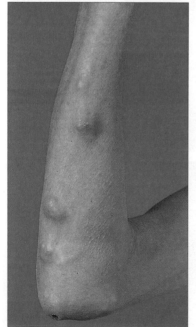

108 Rheumatoid nodules. The upper forearm and elbow are the most common sites for skin nodules in rheumatoid arthritis. These nodules result from vasculitis, and they may ulcerate or become necrotic.

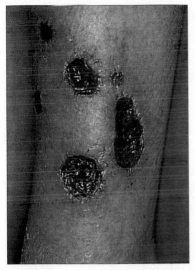

109 Deep arterial ulceration of the legs in rheumatoid arthritis results from vasculitis and is often very difficult to treat.

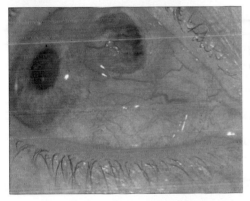

110 Scleromalacia perforans in rheumatoid arthritis. Long-standing inflammation of the sclera (scleritis) has resulted in thinning, which exposes the underlying choroid to secondary infection and the risk of eyeball perforation.

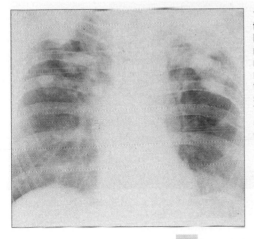

111 Multiple rheumatoid nodules in the lung. These nodules are more common in men, may cavitate and may require further investigation to exclude the possibility of malignancy. This film also shows some rheumatoid fibrotic changes.

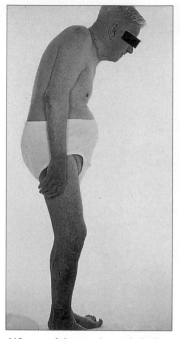 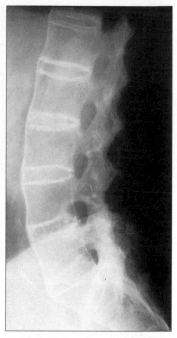

112 Advanced ankylosing spondylitis. Eventually, the trunk may become fixed in a fully bent position, so that the patient cannot see directly ahead – the classic 'question mark' posture.

113 'Bamboo spine'. This lateral X-ray of the lumbar spine in advanced ankylosing spondylitis shows rigid ankylosis resulting from calcification of the spinal ligaments.

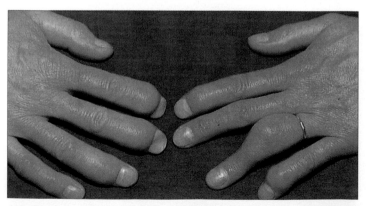

114 Psoriatic arthritis involving mainly the distal interphalangeal joints. There is also deformity and swelling of the left fourth proximal interphalangeal joint (dactylitis).

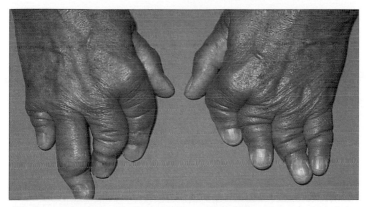

115 Severe psoriatic arthritis (arthritis mutilans). The phalanges have 'telescoped', resulting in shortening of the fingers and gross impairment of function.

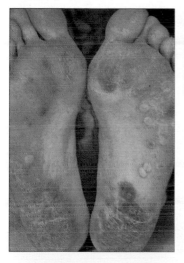

116 Keratoderma blenorrhagicum in Reiter's syndrome. The hyperkeratotic patches coalesce into raised yellow-brown patches. They are typically found on the soles of the feet but may be found in all skin areas. Pustular psoriasis may produce the same features.

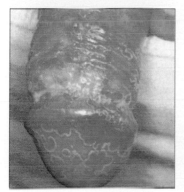

117 Circinate balanitis in Reiter's syndrome. Small, discrete, round or oval red macules or erosions often become confluent.

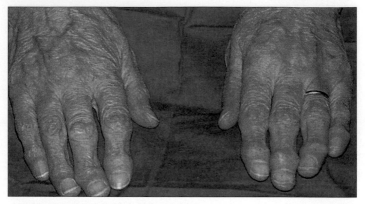

118 Osteoarthritis of the hands showing Heberden's nodes at the distal interphalangeal joints and Bouchard's nodes at the proximal interphalangeal joints.

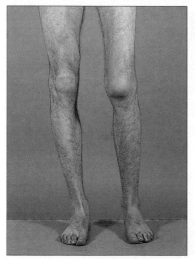

119 Bilateral osteoarthritis of the knees, associated with joint deformity, an effusion (confirmed clinically) in the patient's left knee and severe wasting of the quadriceps muscles in both thighs.

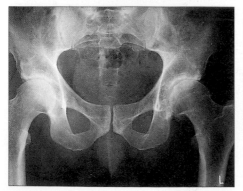

120 Osteoarthritis of the left hip. Note irregular narrowing of the joint space, thinning of the cartilage, osteophytes (projections of new bone) and generalized thinning of the bone in the left femoral head, with early bone cyst formation. The right hip is normal.

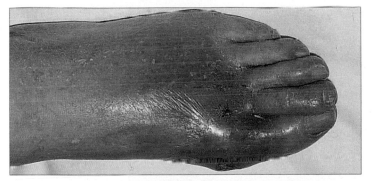

121 Gout. A classic attack of gout affects the big toe.

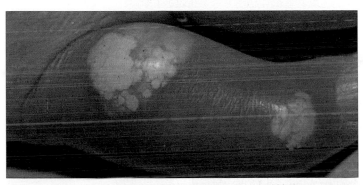

122 'Acute on chronic' gout in the little finger. The tophi helped to confirm the diagnosis. On aspiration, they were found to contain urate crystals.

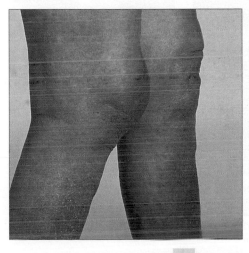

123 Tuberculous effusion of the right knee. In this patient, arthritis followed untreated pulmonary tuberculosis. The knee joint was destroyed. Note also the signs of weight loss in the legs.

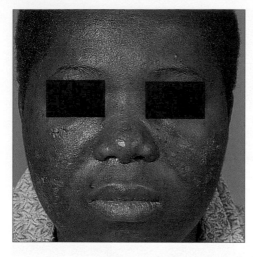

124 Systemic lupus erythematosus is most common in black women of child-bearing age, such as this 33-year-old West Indian woman who presented with a rash over her cheeks.

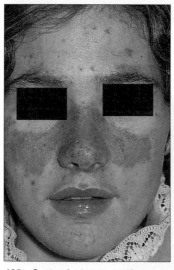

125 Systemic lupus erythematosus. The classic bat or butterfly wing rash in a 17-year-old white. The rash was accompanied by fever, weight loss and polyarthropathy.

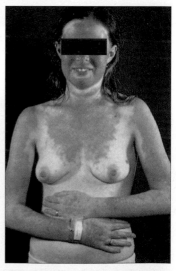

126 Systemic lupus erythematosus. A persistent erythematous rash may occur in sun-exposed areas.

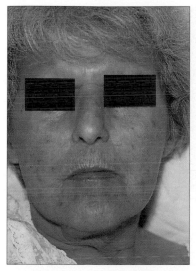

127 Systemic sclerosis. Puckering of the perioral skin is seen; the skin is generally waxy and shiny, and multiple telangiectasia are visible on the face and neck.

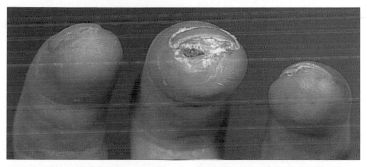

128 In the calcinosis of systemic sclerosis the calcium deposits are characteristically seen in the fingers. Here, they have ulcerated through the skin.

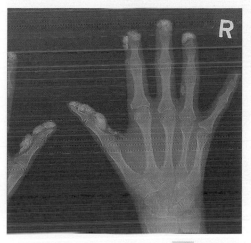

129 Systemic sclerosis. X-ray examination may show extensive calcinosis even in the absence of marked ulceration.

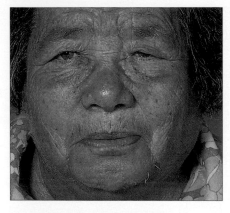

130 Dermatomyositis. This elderly lady has characteristic erythema and oedema of the face. She also complained of proximal muscle weakness. Investigation revealed that she had an underlying carcinoma of the bronchus.

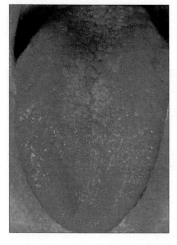

131 Sjögren's syndrome. A bone-dry tongue (xerostomia) results from the involvement of the salivary glands.

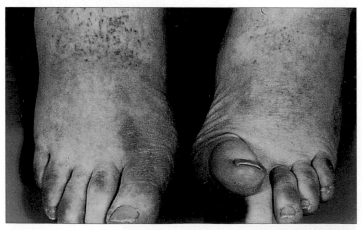

132 Polyarteritis nodosa. There is a vasculitic purpuric rash over the dorsum of both feet and the patient has a mononeuritis – he is unable to dorsiflex his right toe.

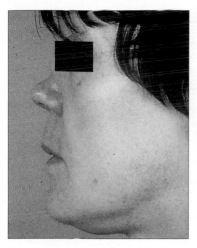

133 Wegener's granulomatosis. The classic appearance after collapse of the nasal septum resulting from granulomatous infiltration.

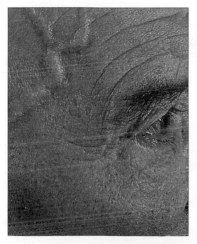

134 Temporal arteritis. The right temporal artery is dilated in this 74-year-old man who had severe headache, burning and tenderness over the artery and visual disturbance. Biopsy was diagnostic.

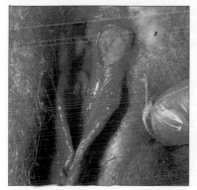

135   Behçet's syndrome. Ulceration of the labium minus was accompanied by ulceration of the lips and uveitis.

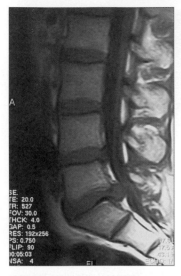

136 Prolapsed intervertebral disc. MRI scan shows a large disc protrusion at the L5/S1 level, with resultant compression of the right S1 nerve root.

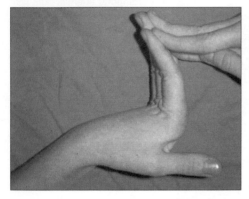

137 Ehlers–Danlos syndrome, showing extreme extensibility of the fingers, which was associated with hyper-elasticity of the skin.

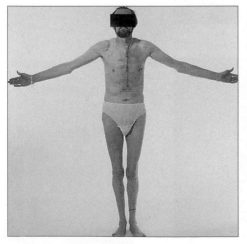

138 Marfan syndrome is an autosomal dominant condition, characterized by tall stature, reduced upper segment to lower segment ratio, long fingers and toes. It is commonly associated with laxity of the joints, a high arched palate, dislocation of the lens, dissecting aneurysm of the aorta, aortic regurgitation and a floppy mitral valve.

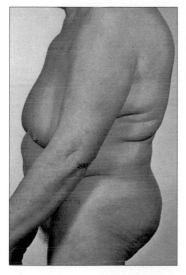

139 Osteoporosis results in vertebral collapse with loss of height associated with chronic backache, bouts of severe back pain and kyphosis (dowager's hump). Creases often appear in the skin, and the ribs may rub on the iliac crest.

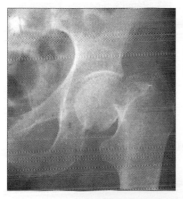

140 Osteoporosis is the usual underlying disorder In fracture of the neck of the femur in the elderly. This patient has a subcapital fracture, which may lead to osteonecrosis of the femoral head.

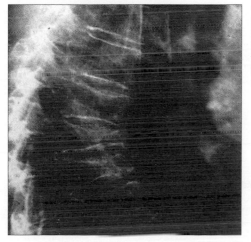

141 Osteoporosis leads to vertebral collapse. This radiograph shows wedge-shaped flattening of the vertebral bodies in the midthoracic region.

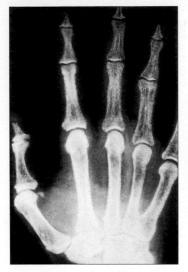

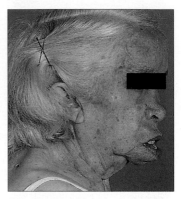

142 Hyperparathyroidism. There are subperiosteal erosions along the cortical surfaces of the middle and distal phalanges, especially obvious in the index finger, and gross resorption of the distal phalanges.

143 Paget's disease. Frontal bossing of the skull leads to a distorted facial appearance. This patient has gross changes and she presented with deafness secondary to ossicular involvement.

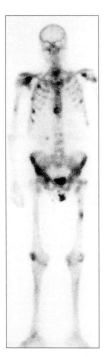

144 Multiple bone metastases are seen in this 99mTc-MDP bone scintigram of a 46-year-old woman with lung cancer. A similar appearance may occur with other metastases, for example from tumours of the breast or kidney.

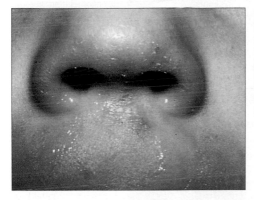

145 The common cold is the most common respiratory disorder. Nasal discharge contains viruses that may spread from person to person in droplets disseminated by sneezing or by direct contact.

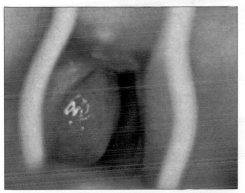

146 Allergic rhinitis is another common upper respiratory disorder, which is associated with a greyish appearance in the nasal mucous membrane, especially when chronic.

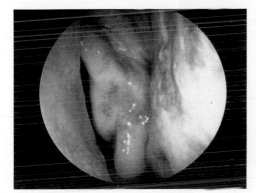

147 Nasal polyps, viewed endoscopically. Nasal polyposis is a relatively frequent accompaniment of asthma and is particularly common in adult asthmatics with sensitivity to aspirin.

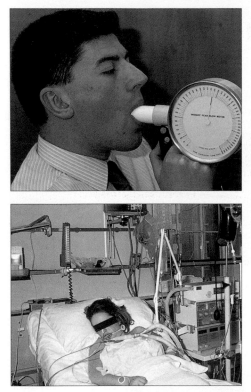

148 & 149 The range of presentation of asthma. The patient in **148** was found incidentally to have a degree of reversible airways obstruction during a medical examination for other reasons. He had never been aware of symptoms. The patient in **149**, by comparison, presented as a medical emergency with acute severe breathlessness and required immediate intensive care including intermittent positive-pressure ventilation.

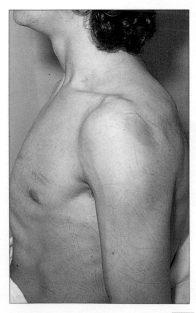

150 Barrel-shaped chest in a patient with chronic asthma. The hyperinflation results from air-trapping in the lungs. Note the associated indrawing of the intercostal muscles.

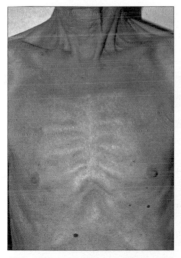

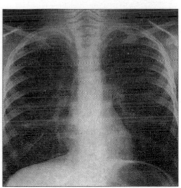

151 Dyspnoea in a patient with severe asthma. Note the contraction of the accessory muscles of respiration.

152 The chest X-ray is a poor guide to the severity of asthma. Although this patient had acute severe asthma requiring urgent treatment, his chest X-ray showed only mild hyperinflation with horizontally aligned ribs.

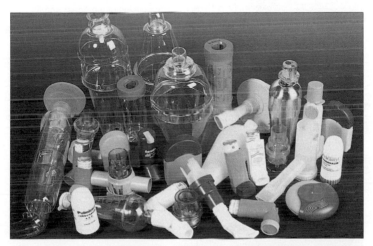

153 Inhaler devices in asthma. This picture includes various pressurized metered-dose inhalers, spacer devices, dry powder inhalers and nebulizer chambers.

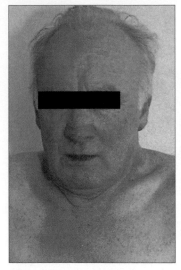

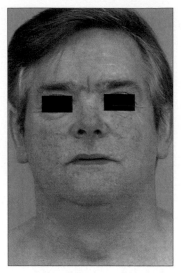

154 Chronic obstructive pulmonary disease (COPD) – a 'pink puffer'. Some patients with severe long-standing COPD have a well maintained PaO_2 and a low $PaCO_2$. These patients are not cyanosed but are breathless, hence the term 'pink puffer.'

155 COPD – a 'blue bloater'. In these patients, the $PaCO_2$ has risen, and the PaO_2 has fallen. Breathlessness at rest is not prominent, and the patient looks more comfortable than the 'pink puffer'. 'Blue bloaters' have right heart failure, and the combination of cyanosis and peripheral oedema accounts for the term.

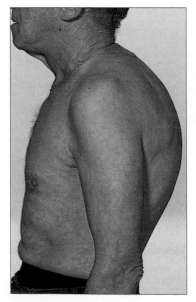

156 COPD – emphysema. The hyperinflation of the chest and associated kyphosis are typical but not diagnostic. A similar appearance may be seen in any chronic respiratory disorder. Note the 'pursed lip' appearance.

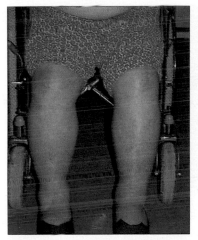

157 COPD with right heart failure causing gross peripheral oedema. The patient was a typical 'blue bloater' and he was not unduly breathless.

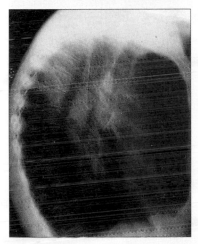

158 COPD – emphysema There is hyperinflation of the chest with sparse lung markings, a marked increase in the posteroanterior diameter of the chest, and diaphragmatic depression. Hilar calcification resulting from old, healed tuberculosis is also well seen in this patient.

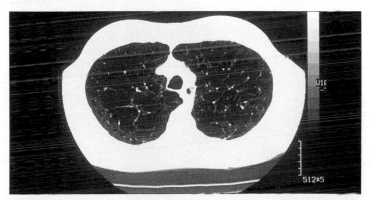

159 CT scan of emphysema. Bullous areas and reduced density of the lung structure are well shown on thin slices of lung in a CT scan.

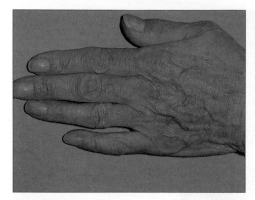

160 Respiratory acidosis produces peripheral vasodilatation, giving hands which are warm, dry and cyanosed. A bounding pulse and tachycardia are common, with dilatation of the peripheral veins. A flapping tremor of the hands may also develop.

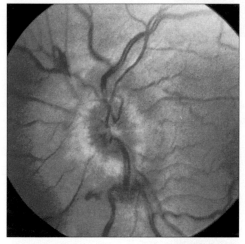

161 Papilloedema occurs in respiratory failure as a result of the increased cerebral and retinal blood flow caused by CO_2 retention.

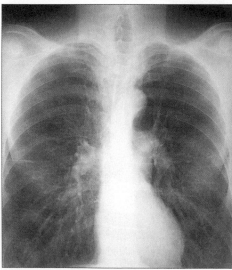

162 Cor pulmonale in a patient with COPD. Both pulmonary arteries are enlarged, and there is marked peripheral pruning of the pulmonary vessels. There is also a small pleural effusion on the right in the horizontal fissure.

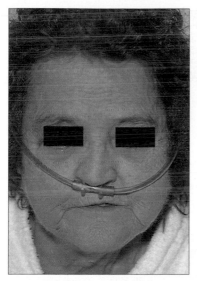

163 Long-term oxygen therapy from cylinders or an oxygen concentrator may be of value in patients with chronic stable respiratory failure. The flow rate and concentration are adjusted to relieve arterial hypoxaemia while avoiding carbon dioxide narcosis.

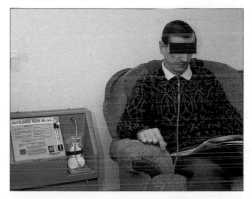

164 An oxygen concentrator in use. These devices are driven by mains electricity and can deliver oxygen in concentrations of 93% or higher at a flow rate of 2–3 litres/minute.

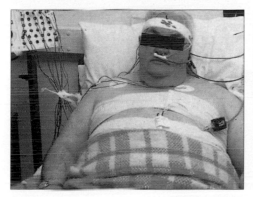

165 Sleep apnoea under investigation in a sleep laboratory. The syndrome should always be considered in patients with chronic respiratory disease who complain of daytime somnolence, or whose partners complain about the patient's snoring or apnoeic episodes at night.

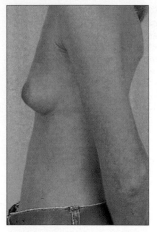

166 Cystic fibrosis presenting at the age of 18 years. This girl had previously been diagnosed as asthmatic, but she presented with weight loss (note the loose trousers and belt), and a sweat test confirmed the diagnosis.

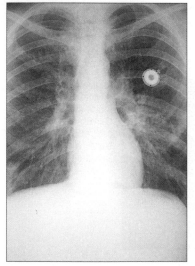

167 Cystic fibrosis. Widespread bronchiectatic changes are present, with an area of consolidation at the right costophrenic angle representing acute infection. An indwelling intravenous catheter for antibiotic administration is present.

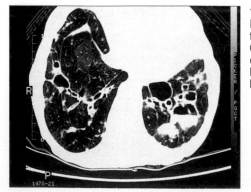

168 Bronchiectasis. Florid cystic bronchiectasis demonstrated on CT scanning. Fluid levels are present in grossly dilated lower lobe bronchi.

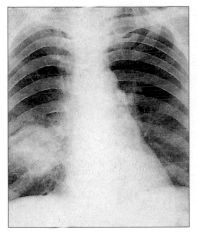

169 Staphylococcal lung abscess in the right lung of an intravenous drug misuser. The abscess is in the lower zone, and a lateral film showed it was in the middle lobe of the lung. Note that there is also extensive calcification of the left hilum, which results from healed tuberculosis.

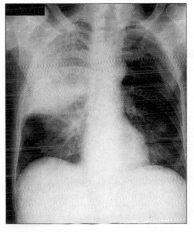

170 Pneumonia. The consolidation involves the whole of the right upper lobe, and a small amount of fluid is present in the horizontal fissure. There are also some areas of consolidation in the right and left lower zones.

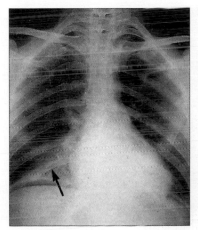

171 Postoperative pneumonia is common after abdominal surgery. Note the gas shadows below both diaphragms. There is right basal consolidation, which results from a combination of aspiration and poor chest movement postoperatively. A typical air bronchogram is arrowed.

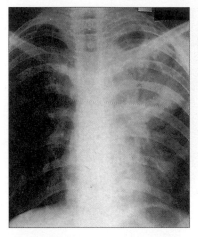

172 Tuberculous left upper zone pneumonia, confirmed by sputum examination. The presence of an air bronchogram in the left upper zone confirms that the underlying pathology is consolidation rather than collapse.

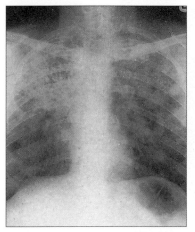

173 Active tuberculosis. This film shows multiple areas of shadowing, especially in the upper lobes, and several lesions have started to cavitate.

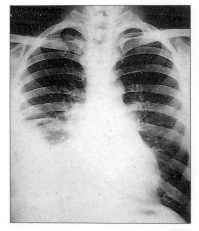

174 Tuberculous pleural effusion. This patient presented with a 6-month history of malaise and weight loss. The large right pleural effusion is accompanied by fluid in the horizontal fissure. Aspiration and culture confirmed the diagnosis.

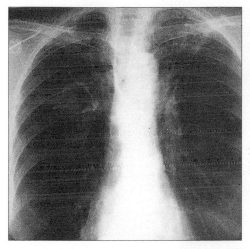

175 Bilateral apical fibrosis resulting from pulmonary tuberculosis. The hila are elevated, and streaky linear shadows extend from the hila to the apices. Scattered calcified upper zone nodules are also present bilaterally.

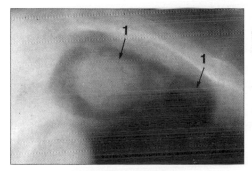

176 Tuberculous cavities containing aspergillomas at the left apex. Tomography clearly demonstrates the round mycetomas or fungus balls (1) within the chronic tuberculous cavities.

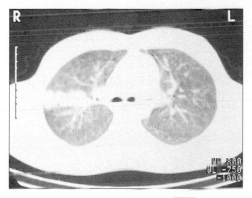

177 Tuberculous pneumonic consolidation and hilar node enlargement demonstrated by CT scan. The consolidation can be seen to extend from the hilum to the pleura.

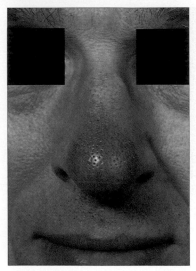

178 Sarcoidosis. Lupus pernio is the term used to describe a dusky-purple infiltration of the skin of the nose in chronic sarcoidosis.

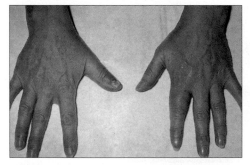

179 Sarcoidosis. The left index finger shows obvious signs of inflammation and swelling (dactylitis), particularly of the proximal phalanx and interphalangeal joint, and the other digits are also involved.

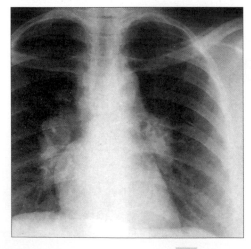

180 Sarcoidosis. There is bilateral hilar lymphadenopathy (1), with increased right paratracheal shadowing (2) and shadowing in the aorticopulmonary window (3).

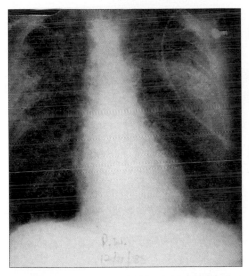

181 Adult respiratory distress syndrome. The chest X-ray appearances in this portable anteroposterior (AP) film are similar to those seen in cardiogenic pulmonary oedema, but the condition results from an increase in pulmonary capillary permeability rather than from heart failure.

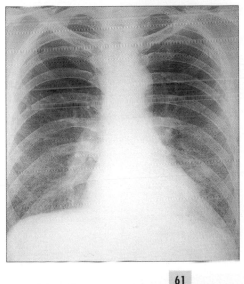

182 Cryptogenic fibrosing alveolitis – gross clubbing of the fingers is common. Note also the tar staining of the fingers in this patient who continued to smoke despite his precarious respiratory state.

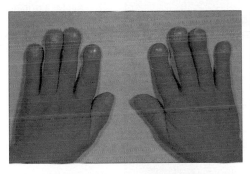

183 Cryptogenic fibrosing alveolitis typically causes predominantly basal pulmonary shadowing. The appearance is very similar to that found in rheumatoid fibrosis.

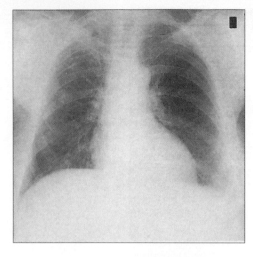

184 Radiation fibrosis following right mastectomy and radiotherapy. There are fibrotic changes in the lung, with upper lobe shrinkage, especially on the right, and the trachea is pulled to the right. There are also some ununited rib fractures on the right, resulting from secondary deposits.

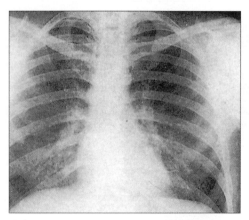

185 Acute extrinsic allergic alveolitis – in this case pigeon fancier's lung. The X-ray shows diffuse, hazy opacification in both lung fields, which partially obscures the normal vascular markings.

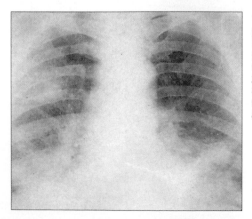

186 Complicated pneumoconiosis. Large irregular fibrotic masses are present, mainly in both lower zones and on the right. Similar appearances may occur in complicated silicosis.

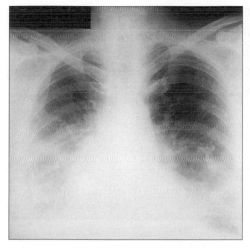

187 Asbestosis. The advanced fibrotic changes in the lungs are best seen around the heart and in the lower zones. The patient's occupational exposure was as a shipyard worker.

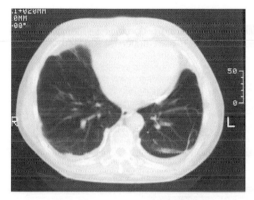

188 CT scan in asbestosis. There are widespread fibrotic changes in both lungs and some patchy pleural calcification is seen.

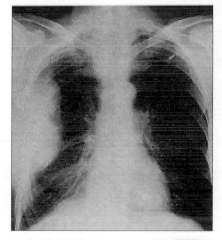

189 Mesothelioma of the right pleura. The patient had a long history of asbestos exposure and has a large pleural mass.

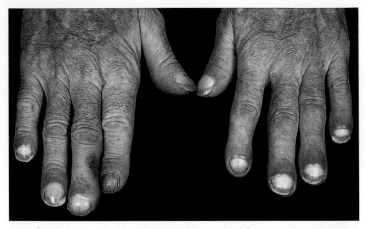

190 Carcinoma of the bronchus, with tar-stained fingers and acute, recent onset clubbing (note the reddening and swelling of the nailfolds). The patient smoked 40 cigarettes/day and had bronchial carcinoma.

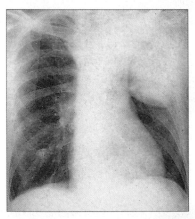

191 Carcinoma of the bronchus– left upper lobe opacity. Much of the shadowing is the result of infection and collapse of the lung distal to the point at which the tumour causes bronchial obstruction. Note the extensive calcification in the right hilum and lower zone – the result of healed tuberculosis.

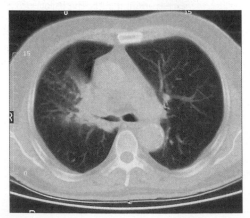

192 Bronchial carcinoma on CT scan, surrounding and narrowing the right upper lobe bronchus, with obstructive changes peripheral to it. Note the incidental presence of calcification in the wall of the descending aorta.

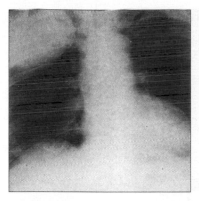

193 Right apical carcinoma of the bronchus (Pancoast tumour). In this location, the tumour may cause other symptoms and signs, including Horner's syndrome and wasting of the small muscles of the hands.

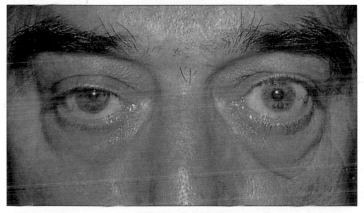

194 Horner's syndrome resulting from a right Pancoast tumour. The patient had a right ptosis and a constricted right pupil, caused by tumour infiltration of the inferior cervical sympathetic ganglia.

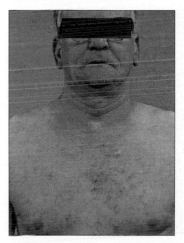

195 Superior vena caval obstruction in bronchial carcinoma. Note the swelling of the head and neck, engorgement of the neck veins and the development of a collateral circulation in the veins of the chest wall.

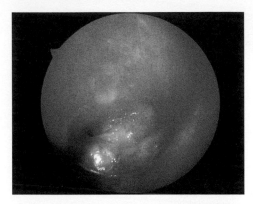

196 Left upper lobe bronchial carcinoma seen on bronchoscopy.

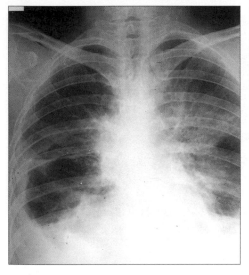

197 Lymphangitis carcinomatosa. Micronodular shadows are seen throughout the lungs and there is tumour infiltration of lymphatic vessels.

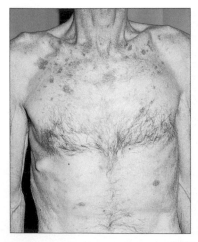

198 Multiple secondary deposits in the skin in a patient with carcinoma of the bronchus. Note the signs of weight loss and the subcutaneous nodule on the right.

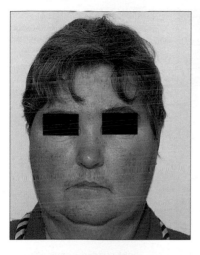

199 Cushing's syndrome resulting from ectopic adrenocoticotrophin hormone (ACTH) secretion by a small-cell bronchial carcinoma. The disease often runs a very rapid course.

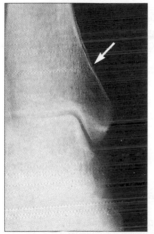

200 Hypertrophic pulmonary osteoarthropathy (HPOA) at the ankle in a patient with bronchial carcinoma. New bone formation is shown by the double margin seen at the medial border of the tibia (arrowed).

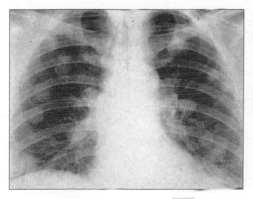

201 Cannonball metastases in both lung fields. Secondary lung deposits occur with a number of tumours, including those of the kidney, ovary, breast, pancreas and testicle, and also malignant melanoma.

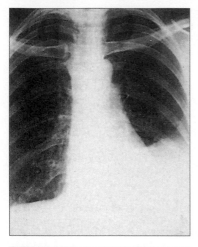

202 Left pleural effusion, which was associated with fever and pleuritic pain and resulted from infection in this patient.

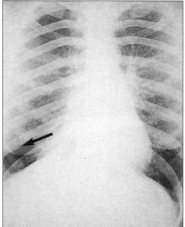

203 Right – sided pneumothorax in an adult woman with asthma. The edge of the collapsed lung is marked with an arrow. It is important to consider pneumothorax whenever examining the chest X-ray of a patient with an acute respiratory problem.

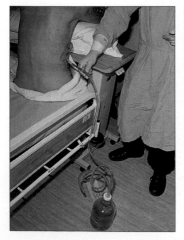

204 An intercostal drain. The chosen insertion site is the 6th intercostal space and the drainage tube can be attached to a one-way valve or, as here, to an underwater seal drain.

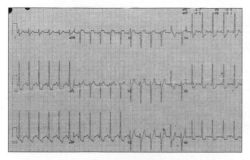

205 Angina pectoris associated with ECG changes. This ECG was taken during an episode of exercise-induced angina, and it shows ST-segment depression (4 mm) in leads V4–6, standard leads II and III and lead aVF.

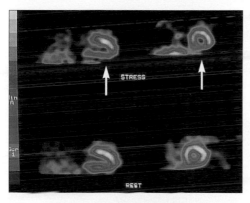

206 Impaired myocardial perfusion demonstrated by nuclear tomography. During exercise (stress), the inferior wall of the left ventricle is poorly perfused, as shown in the ventricular long axis (top left) and short axis (top right) views (arrows). After rest, a greater though still abnormally low level of perfusion is seen.

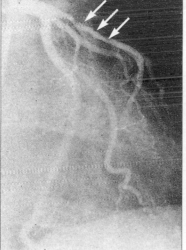

207 A left anterior descending coronary artery stricture, demonstrated by coronary angiography (arrows).

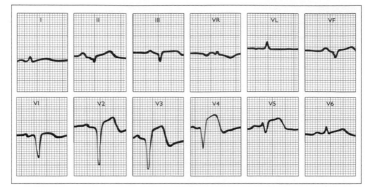

208 Acute anterior myocardial infarction extending inferiorly – 3 hours after onset. The changes are those of acute full-thickness infarction, with widespread ST-segment and T-wave changes and Q waves in V1–V4.

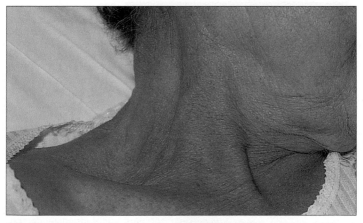

209 Elevated external jugular venous pressure (JVP) suggested right heart failure in this patient following myocardial infarction.

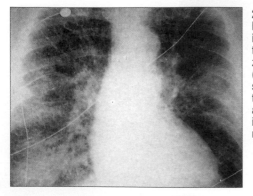

210 Heart failure following myocardial infarction. There is distension of the upper zone vessels, interstitial (Kerley B) lines are present at both bases; and there are some areas of apparent consolidation, indicating alveolar pulmonary oedema.

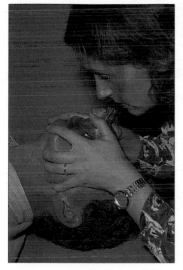

211 Cardiac arrest. Artificial respiration via a Laerdal mask. The movement of the chest provides an index of the efficacy of ventilation.

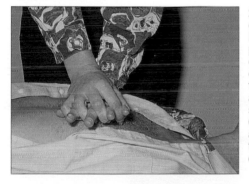

212 Cardiac arrest: cardiac massage. The heel of one hand is placed on the lower third of the sternum and the other hand is rested on top of the first with the arms straight. Using a sharp jerky movement, 60–90 strokes per minute are administered, aiming to move the sternum 3–5 cm at each stroke.

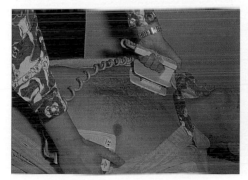

213 Cardiac arrest: external DC defibrillation should be performed if the heart has not restarted or the ECG shows ventricular fibrillation, or both. The electrodes must be well separated to avoid a short circuit, electrolyte jelly is necessary for good contact with the skin, and all personnel should stand clear of the patient to avoid receiving an electric shock.

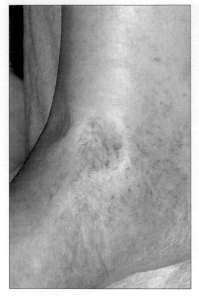

214 Pitting oedema in cardiac failure following myocardial infarction. A depression ('pit') remains in the oedema for some minutes after firm fingertip pressure is applied.

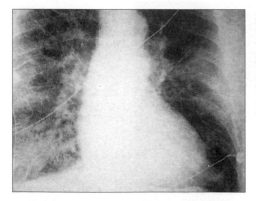

215 Ventricular aneurysm, 3 weeks after acute myocardial infarction. Note the bulge in the left cardiac border. On screening, this was found to move paradoxically outwards during systole.

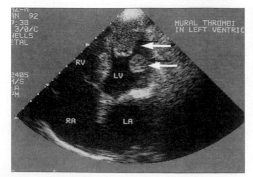

216 Left ventricular thrombus after myocardial infarction. The diastolic apical four-chamber view shows at least two large thrombi on the apical and anterior walls of the left ventricle (arrowed).

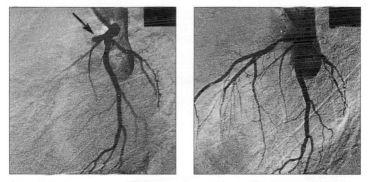

217 & 218 Coronary angiography and angioplasty. The coronary angiogram in left lateral projection shows complete occlusion of the left anterior descending coronary artery. Only a stump is seen (arrow). After coronary angioplasty there is good perfusion of the left anterior descending artery, although a residual stenosis is seen (**218**). This can, if necessary, be dealt with electively at a later stage by further angioplasty, stenting or surgery.

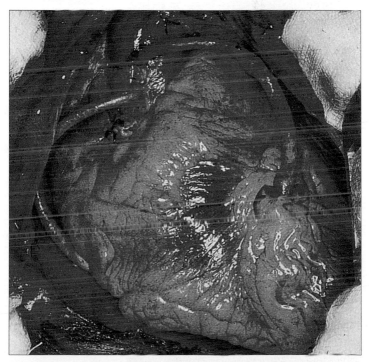

219 Coronary artery surgery. Bypass grafts to the right and left anterior descending coronary arteries are in position.

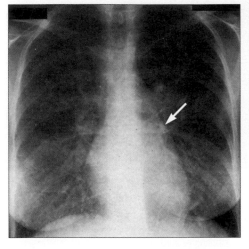

220 Mitral stenosis, causing heart failure. The left atrial appendage is enlarged (arrowed), the upper zone blood vessels are distended and there are linear densities in the periphery of the lower zones (interstitial or Kerley's B lines).

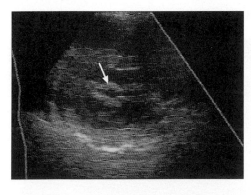

221 Echocardiogram (short-axis view) showing tight mitral stenosis. The tight orifice of the mitral valve is arrowed.

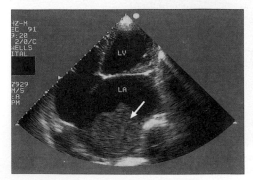

222 Echocardiogram (parasternal short-axis view) in a patient with rheumatic mitral stenosis and atrial fibrillation, showing a very large thrombus attached to the walls of the left atrium (arrow). The patient presented with a stroke.

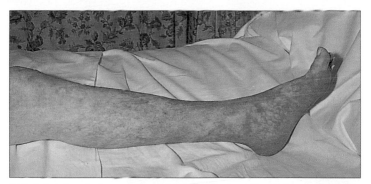

223 Arterial embolism causing acute ischaemia of the leg in a patient with mitral stenosis. The patient was in atrial fibrillation, and the source of the embolus was the left atrium.

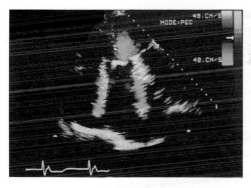

224 Mitral and tricuspid regurgitation shown by colour-flow mapping. The left ventricle is the blue area at the top of the image, and the regurgitant flow through the mitral valve is seen on the right. Tricuspid regurgitation is seen as a narrower band of flow on the left.

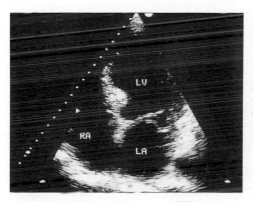

225 Mitral valve prolapse on two-dimensional cardiac ultrasound. The posterior cusp of the mitral valve is seen to prolapse into the left atrium in this systolic frame (LV = left ventricle; LA = left atrium; RA = right atrium).

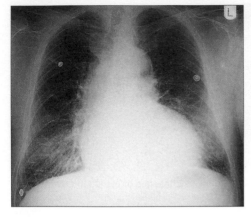

226 Aortic stenosis and heart failure. There is gross cardiomegaly, with a bilateral symmetrical increase in bronchovascular markings, especially in the lower zones. Bilateral Kerley B lines are consistent with pulmonary oedema.

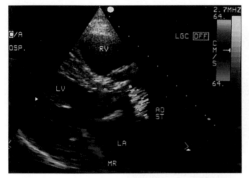

227 Aortic stenosis–colour-flow Doppler mapping. The typical jet flow through the stenotic aortic valve is seen (AO ST), and there is also a minor degree of mitral regurgitation (MR) (RV = right ventricle; LV = left ventricle; LA = left atrium).

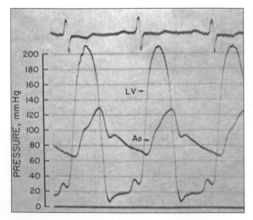

228 Aortic stenosis at cardiac catheterization. Note the low aortic (Ao) pressure compared with the left ventricular pressure (LV) and the delayed peak in aortic pressure – both characteristic of severe aortic stenosis.

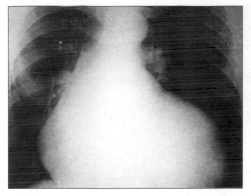

229 Aortic regurgitation leading to left ventricular hypertrophy and dilatation. The left heart border is more convex than normal, and the cardiac enlargement seen here is indicative of ventricular dilatation.

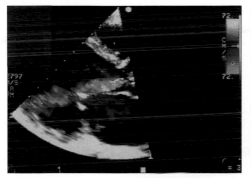

230 Mild aortic regurgitation (parasternal long-axis view). The aortic regurgitant jet (in blue) is directed posteriorly from the aortic valve (to the right in the picture), back into the left ventricle (to the left in the picture), impinging directly on the anterior mitral valve leaflet (in the centre of the picture immediately below the blue jet).

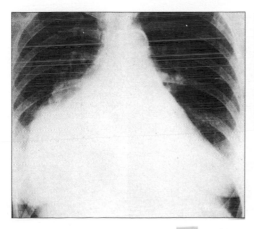

231 Tricuspid regurgitation. The enlargement of the right heart shadow is caused by a grossly enlarged right atrium. Note also the calcified aortic arch (and the incidental bilateral hilar calcification, resulting from old tuberculosis).

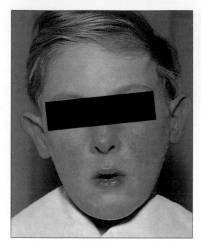

232 Fallot's tetralogy is the most common cause of cyanotic congenital heart disease in patients over the age of 1 year. This boy has severe central cyanosis.

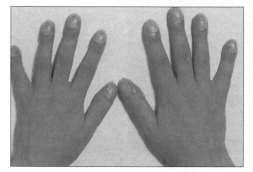

233 Severe finger clubbing in a patient with cyanotic congenital heart disease. The nailbeds are obviously cyanotic.

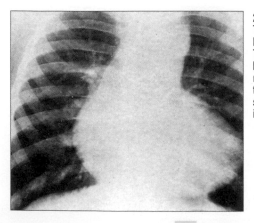

234 Fallot's tetralogy. The classic boot-shaped heart (coeur-en-sabot). The appearance is brought about by gross right ventricular hypertrophy, associated with small pulmonary arteries.

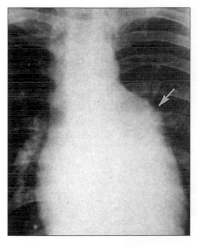

235 Atrial septal defect with a large left-to-right shunt. The pulmonary arteries are prominent, especially on the left (arrow).

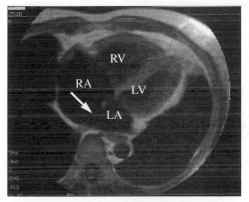

236 Atrial septal defect. This MRI shows an ostium secundum atrial septal defect (arrow). The right ventricle and right atrium are dilated (RA = right atrium; RV = right ventricle; LA = left atrium; LV = left ventricle).

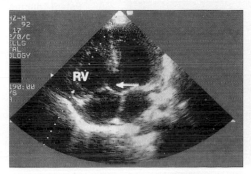

237 Ventricular septal defect (arrowed) in an apical four-chamber echocardiogram. There is also enlargement of the right ventricle (RV) due to the left-to-right shunt.

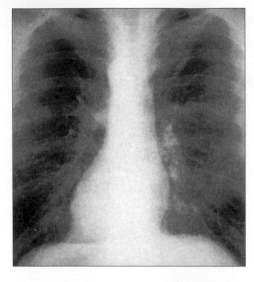

238 Situs inversus revealed by chest X-ray. The apex of the heart lies in the right side of the thorax (dextrocardia). The left dome of the diaphragm is higher than the right, because the liver is on the left and the spleen and the stomach are on the right.

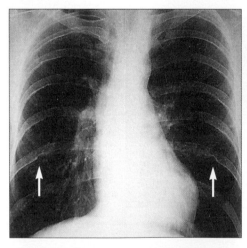

239 Coarctation of the aorta. There is bilateral rib notching as a result of dilated intercostal arteries, e.g. in both 8th ribs (arrows). This 30-year-old man presented with hypertension.

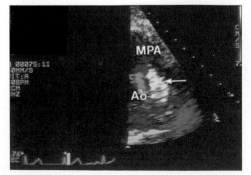

240 Patent ductus arteriosus. This colour-flow Doppler (short-axis view) shows a characteristic ductal jet (arrowed), which represents flow from the aorta (Ao) into the main pulmonary artery (MPA).

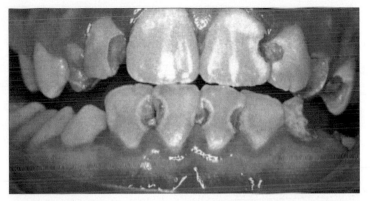

241 Severe dental caries and gingivitis predisposes patients to episodes of bacteraemia, and thus to infective endocarditis in the presence of a congenital or acquired heart abnormality.

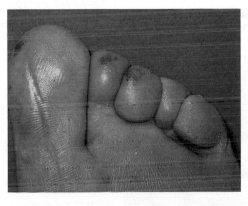

242 Small dermal infarcts in infective endocarditis. These infarcts are usually tender. They may be caused by septic emboli from the cardiac vegetations or by vasculitis.

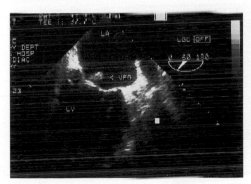

243 Transoesophageal echocardiography is a valuable technique for demonstrating cardiac vegetations in infective endocarditis. Here a vegetation attached to the atrial surface of the mitral valve is clearly seen.

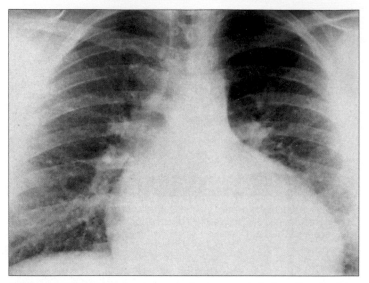

244 Acute myocarditis causing marked enlargement of all cardiac chambers and pulmonary venous congestion. An identical chest X-ray appearance may be seen in dilated cardiomyopathy.

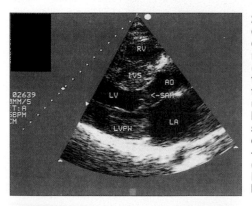

245 Hypertrophic obstructive cardiomyopathy. The left ventricle posterior wall (LVPW) is thickened, and there is hypertrophy of the inter-ventricular septum (IVS). As blood leaves the left ventricle it sucks the anterior leaflet of the mitral valve forward – systolic anterior motion (SAM) (LA = left atrium; RV = right ventricle; LV = left ventricle)

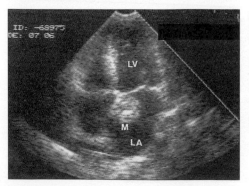

246 Left atrial myxoma. This apical four-chamber echocardiogram shows a circular mass (M) arising in a typical position from the interatrial septum just above the mitral valve (LA = left atrium; LV = left ventricle).

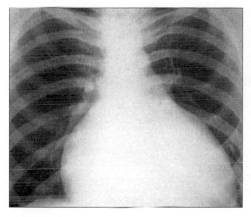

247 Pericardial effusion. The heart shadow appears generally enlarged, but the appearance is not diagnostic. A similar appearance can be seen in cardiac failure, in myocarditis or in dilated cardiomyopathy.

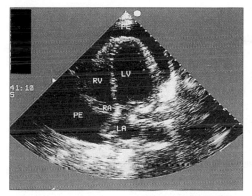

248 Pericardial effusion in carcinoma of the breast. The apical PE indicates a pericardial effusion, whereas that to the left indicates a pleural effusion. In addition there is a solid tissue mass invading the wall of the left atrium and ventricle, which probably represents secondary tumour (LV = left ventricle; RV = right ventricle; LA = left atrium; RA = right atrium).

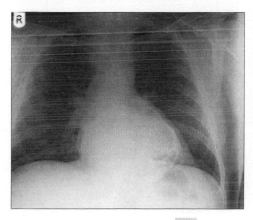

249 Pericardial calcification is clearly seen around the left and inferior borders of the heart. This patient has a normal-sized heart, but the calcification may progress further, leading to constrictive pericarditis.

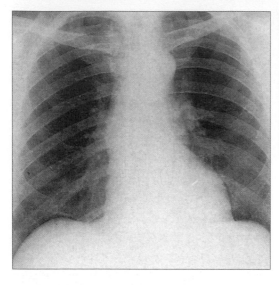

250 Hypertension. The chest X-ray is usually normal in mild to moderate hypertension (as here), but cardiac enlargement associated with left ventricular hypertrophy may occur in the later stages.

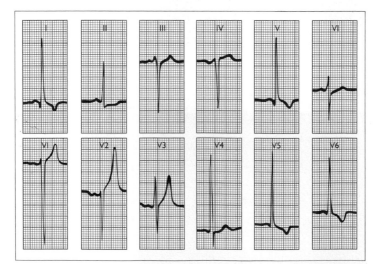

251 Left ventricular hypertrophy in hypertension. Left ventricular hypertrophy (LVH) is present when the R wave in V5 or V6 or the S wave in V1 or V2 exceeds 25 mm in an adult of normal build. This ECG shows severe hypertrophy with T-wave inversion over the left ventricle (V5–6) and in I and VL.

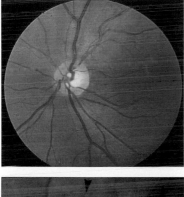

252 – 255 Hypertensive retinopathy is traditionally divided into four grades. Grade 1 (**252**) shows very early and minor changes in a young patient: increased tortuosity of a retinal vessel and increased reflectiveness (silver wiring) of a retinal artery, are seen at 1 o'clock in this view. Otherwise, the fundus is completely normal. Grade 2 (**253**) again shows increased tortuosity and silver wiring (coarse arrows). In addition there is 'nipping' of the venules at arteriovenous crossings (fine arrow). Grade 3 (**254**) shows the same changes as grade 2 plus flame-shaped retinal haemorrhages and soft 'cotton-wool' exudates. In Grade 4 (**255**) there is swelling of the optic disc (papilloedema), retinal oedema is present, and hard exudates may collect around the fovea, producing a typical 'macular star'.

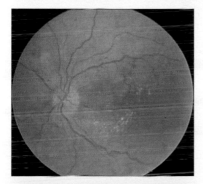

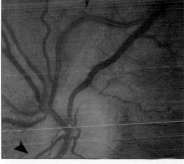

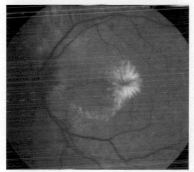

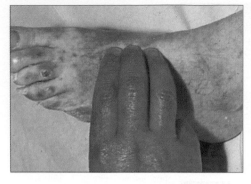

256 Peripheral vascular disease. Typical changes in the skin include atrophy, pallor, loss of hair and, in some patients, trophic nail changes. This patient also has early ulceration on the dorsum of three toes. The dorsalis pedis pulse was impalpable.

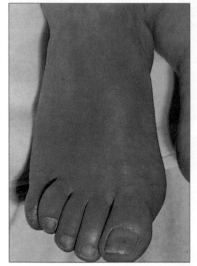

257 'Critical' ischaemia of the foot. The patient had a sudden onset of coldness and loss of sensation in the toes and the dorsum of the foot. He has evidence of chronic ischaemia, including absence of hair and thinness of the skin.

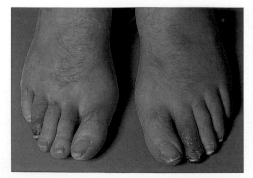

258 Typical dry gangrene of two toes in a patient with diffuse atheroma. Note the chronic nail changes (resembling onycholysis) The residual hair on the dorsum of the feet is unusual in chronic ischaemia.

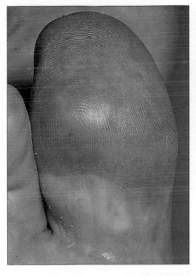

259 Digital ischaemia in Buerger's disease often affects the toes. Here the ischaemia progressed to gangrene, and amputation of the toe was necessary to eliminate infection.

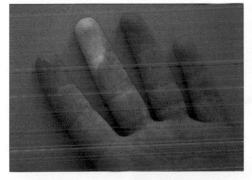

260 Raynaud's syndrome in the acute phase, with severe blanching of the tip of one finger. The phase of pallor is followed by a phase of reactive hyperaemia.

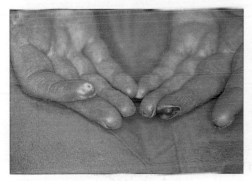

261 Primary Raynaud's syndrome occasionally progresses to fingertip ulceration or gangrene. This 40-year-old woman had small, painful recurrent necrotic ulcers of the fingertips, wasting of the pulps and irregular nail growth.

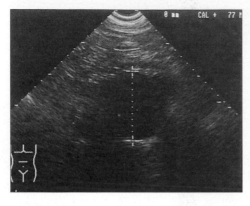

262 Abdominal aortic aneurysm revealed by ultrasound. Echogenic material in the lumen represents layers of thrombus. The diameter of the lumen was 6.2 cm (a diameter over 4 cm is an indication for operative intervention).

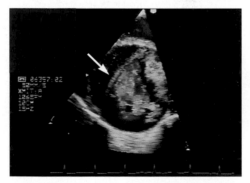

263 Transoesophageal echocardiogram, demonstrating a dissecting aneurysm of the ascending aorta. This view shows a dilated aortic root with an obvious intimal flap (arrowed). There is turbulent blood flow in the true lumen (blue and orange) with no flow in the dissected lumen.

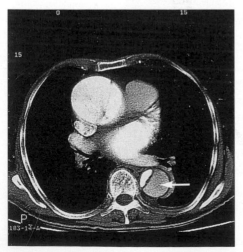

264 Dissecting aneurysm. Contrast-enhanced spiral CT demonstrates dissection of the ascending and descending aorta. In the descending aorta, the true lumen is small, shown white. The 'false lumen' (arrow) is filled with clot.

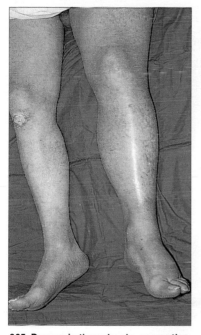

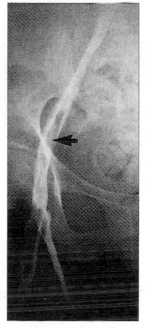

265 Deep vein thrombosis, presenting as an acutely swollen left leg. Note the dilatation of the superficial veins. Less than 50% of DVTs present in this way, and other conditions may mimic DVT, so further investigation is always indicated.

266 Deep vein thrombosis in the iliac vein. Venography is the 'gold standard' in the diagnosis of deep vein thrombosis.

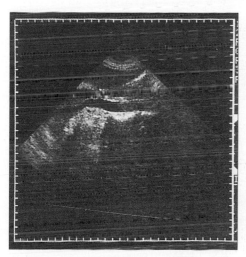

267 Deep vein thrombosis demonstrated by ultrasound. Thrombus can be seen extending from the iliofemoral veins (right of picture) into the inferior vena cava (centre of picture).

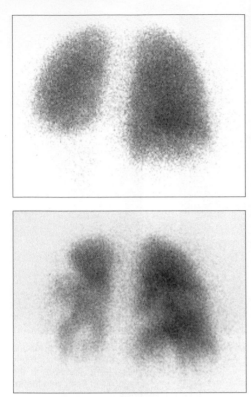

268 & 269 Pulmonary emboli revealed by radionuclide ventilation (268) and perfusion (269) scans. 268 shows a normal distribution of xenon during ventilation, whereas **269** shows multiple perfusion defects in both lung fields when ^{99m}Tc-albumin microspheres were injected. This 'unmatched' perfusion defect is typical of multiple pulmonary emboli.

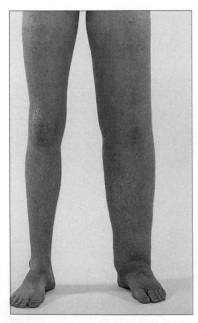

270 Unilateral lymphoedema of unknown cause. Chronic lymphoedema is often more severe above the ankle than below it. The cause in this young man was unknown.

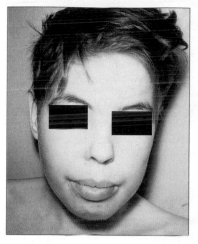

271 Acute nephritis. The generalized facial puffiness and the erythematous periorbital oedema are typical, and this boy also had ankle oedema and hypertension.

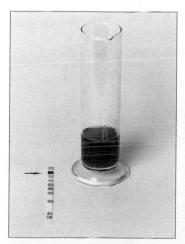

272 A positive result for blood (arrowed) occurred when this reddish-brown urine was tested with a standard stick. The patient had acute nephritis.

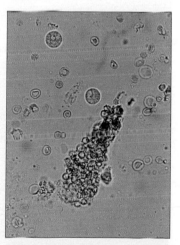

273 A red-cell cast, seen on direct microscopy of urine from a patient with acute nephritis. Red-cell casts imply bleeding at the glomerular level.

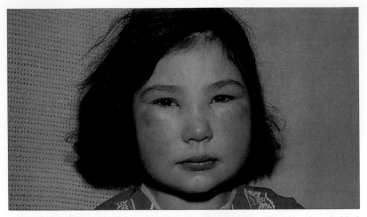

274 Nephrotic syndrome in childhood. Note the gross facial and periorbital oedema, which was associated with gross proteinuria.

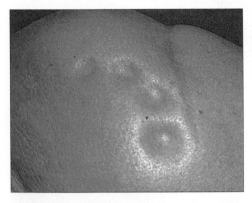

275 Nephrotic syndrome – gross pitting oedema of the abdominal wall, secondary to severe hypoalbuminaemia.

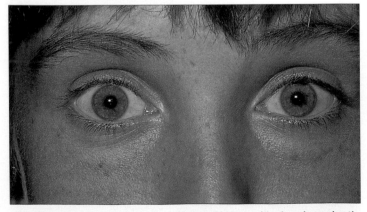

276 Premature corneal arcus in a 15-year-old boy with chronic nephrotic syndrome. This was associated with hypercholesterolaemia and a risk of premature vascular disease.

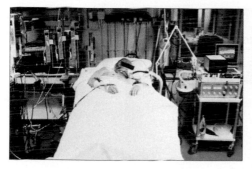

277 Patients with acute renal failure are often severely ill. They commonly require haemodialysis, ventilation and cardiovascular support.

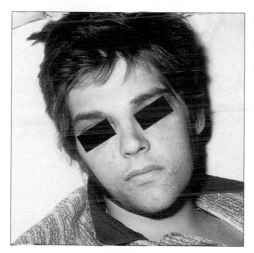

278 Chronic renal failure. Note the pale, sallow, yellow-brown appearance of the skin and the anaemic pallor of the sclerae.

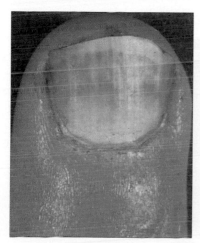

279 The nail in chronic renal failure. Various nail changes may be observed, including discoloration of the distal nail, pallor of the proximal nail and lunula and pigmentation of the skin at the base of the nail.

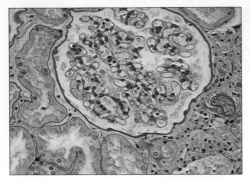

280 A normal glomerulus. (PAS) The light-microscopic appearance of minimal change glomerulonephritis is identical.

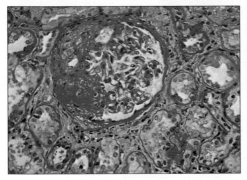

281 Focal and segmental glomerulosclerosis. The segmental sclerosis is clearly seen on the light microscopy of a renal biopsy (PAS). The patient had nephrotic syndrome.

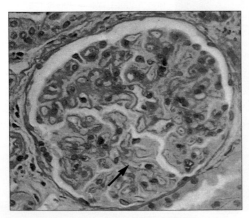

282 Membranous glomerulonephritis. The renal biopsy shows uniform thickening of the capillary basement membranes (arrow). (MSB). This adult patient had nephrotic syndrome.

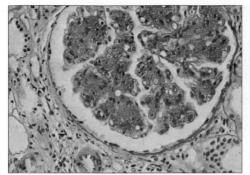

283 Mesangiocapillary glomerulonephritis. There is an increase in mesangial cells and matrix, patchy thickening of the basement membrane and marked lobulation of the glomerular tufts (PAS). The patient presented in renal failure.

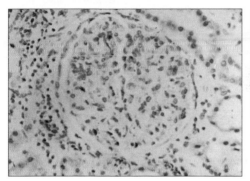

284 Mesangial proliferative glomerulonephritis. There is an increase In mesangial cells and matrix (H & E). The patient had asymptomatic microscopic haematuria and proteinuria.

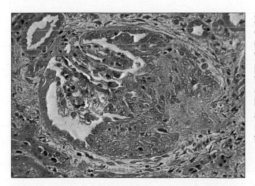

285 Diffuse endocapillary proliferative glomeruloncphritis with a crescent compressing the glomerular tuft (H & E). Crescentic glomerulonephritis may be found in all types of acute nephritis with rapidly progressive renal failure.

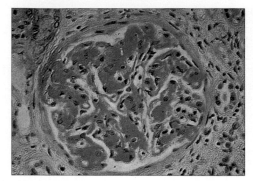

286 Renal amyloidosis. The glomerulus shows amyloid deposition, stained by Congo Red, in the glomerular capillaries.

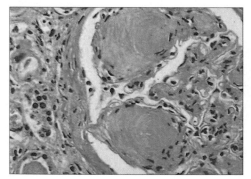

287 Kimmelstiel–Wilson nodules are the classic lesions of diabetic nephropathy. Their presence is virtually diagnostic of diabetes mellitus. Note the nodular intercapillary glomerulosclerosis (MS).

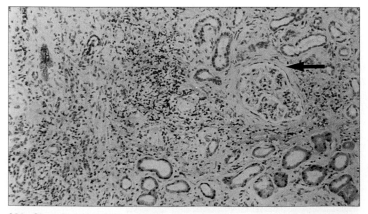

288 Chronic interstitial nephritis. The renal biopsy shows a diffuse lymphocytic infiltrate and fibrosis in the interstisium with focal tubular atrophy and periglomerular scarring (arrow) (H&E).

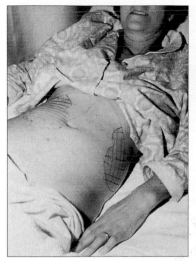

289 Adult polycystic kidney disease. The kidneys are huge and easily palpable as the skin markings show. Cysts are often also present in the liver and pancreas. The patient had chronic renal failure.

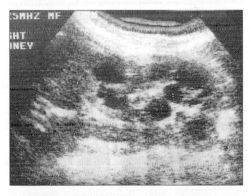

290 Adult polycystic kidneys, shown by ultrasound. The multiple parenchymal cysts are clearly demonstrated.

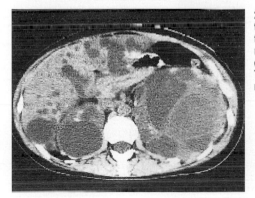

291 Bilateral polycystic kidneys, larger on the patient's left (to the right of the picture), demonstrated by CT. The liver also contains multiple cysts.

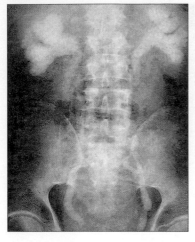

292 Intravenous urogram showing bilateral hydronephrosis and hydro-ureter with a large bladder in an elderly man with chronic urinary retention as a result of prostatic enlargement.

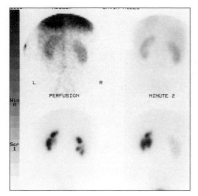

293 99mmTc-DTPA diuretic renogram in a patient with left-sided obstructive uropathy. The patient was given intravenous frusemide (furosemide) at 20 minutes. Isotope persists in the left kidney for much longer than in the normal right kidney.

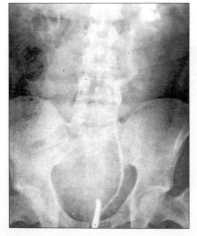

294 Retroperitoneal fibrosis. This condition commonly affects both ureters. Here, the left retrograde ureterogram shows obstruction and distortion of the left ureter and a left hydronephrosis.

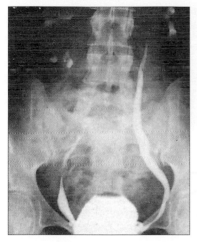

295 Bilateral ureteric reflux, shown on micturating cystogram. There is some ureteric dilatation and early calyceal clubbing, so this is grade III reflux.

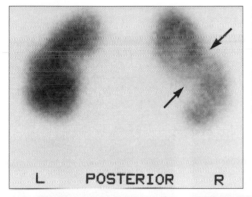

296 Reflux nephropathy with scarring, revealed by 99mTc–DMSA scintigram. The two largest defects are arrowed, but other defects in the right kidney are also evident.

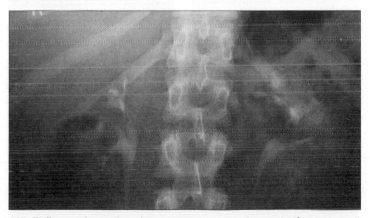

297 Reflux nephropathy – intravenous urogram demonstrating two small contracted kidneys. The cortical scarring and calyceal dilatation and deformity, seen especially in the left upper pole, are typical.

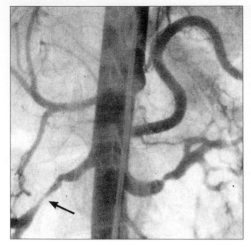

298 Bilateral renal artery stenosis demonstrated by digital subtraction aortography. The appearances are typical of stenosis caused by fibro-muscular hyperplasia rather than atheroma, and the stenosis is more marked on the right (arrow).

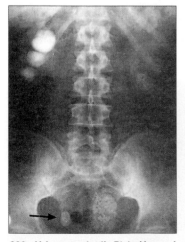

299 Urinary calculi. Plain X-ray of the kidney, ureter and bladder (KUB) shows a rather unusual combination of calculi in both kidneys (more prominent on the right), in the lower right ureter (arrowed) and in a bladder diverticulum.

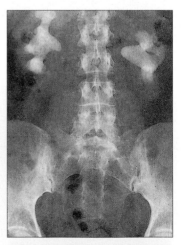

300 Large bilateral staghorn calculi are shown on this plain (KUB) X-ray. The patient presented with recurrent urinary infections.

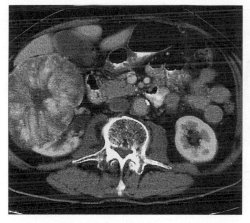

301 Renal cell carcinoma as seen on a contrast CT scan. Compare the massive right renal tumour with the normal kidney seen on the left side.

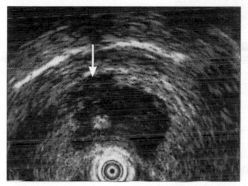

302 A rectal ultrasound probe can be used to define and stage carcinoma of the prostate. The right lobe of the capsule of the prostate is distorted, and anteriorly a capsular breach is evident (arrow), suggesting extracapsular spread of the tumour.

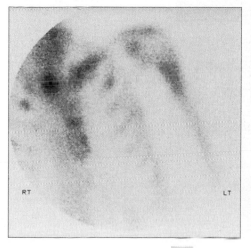

303 Multiple bone metastases in a patient with carcinoma of the prostate, revealed by a bone scintigram. Areas of increased activity are present in the ribs, sternum and left humerus.

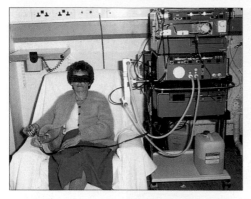

304 Typical patient with chronic renal failure undergoing haemodialysis in a hospital setting. In some countries, many patients carry out this treatment on a long-term basis in a specially converted room at home.

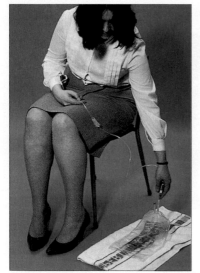

305 Continuous ambulatory peritoneal dialysis (CAPD) is a simpler and less restricting technique than haemodialysis, and is compatible with a virtually normal lifestyle.

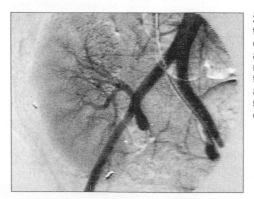

306 Normal renal transplant *in situ*. This digital subtraction angiogram shows the normal site for a renal transplant. The renal artery has been anastomosed to the right external iliac artery.

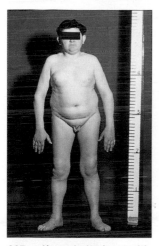

307 Hypopituitarism with gonadotrophin failure in a 39-year-old man. Note the extreme atrophy of the genitalia, the absence of body hair and the apparent gynaecomastia associated with obesity.

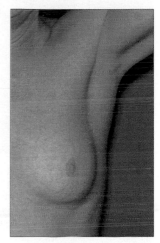

308 Lack of body hair in hypopituitarism. 20 years earlier, this patient developed postpartum pituitary necrosis (Sheehan's syndrome). This resulted in many features of hypopituitarism, including a total absence of axillary and pubic hair.

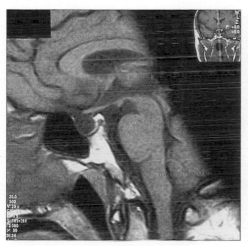

309 Empty sella in a patient with hypopituitarism after postpartum pituitary necrosis, demonstrated by MRI. The pituitary fossa is fluid filled, with no recognizable pituitary tissue.

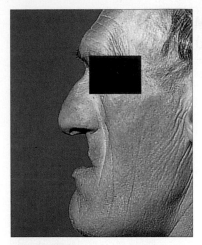

310 Acromegaly. Profile showing prognathism, thickening of the soft tissues and skin, and increased prominence of the supra-orbital ridge and nose.

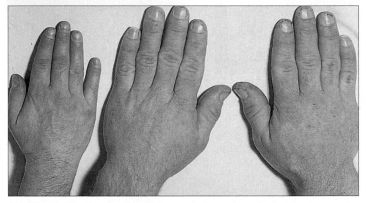

311 Spade-like hands are often an obvious abnormality in acromegaly. Compare the acromegalic hands on the right with the normal hand on the left.

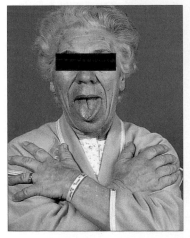

312 Enlargement of the tongue in acromegaly is obvious in this patient, who also shows other facial signs, and has classic changes in her hands.

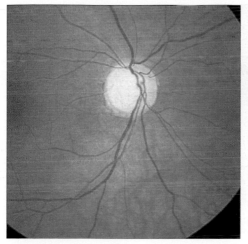

313 Optic atrophy in a patient with acromegaly. The flat, pale optic disc has a well defined margin and the appearance of 'primary' optic atrophy. This type of optic atrophy results from compression of the optic pathways by the tumour.

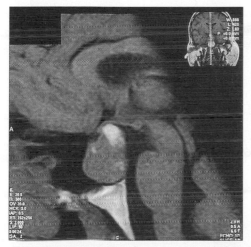
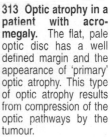

314 Pituitary macroadenoma in acromegaly. A large tumour is demonstrated on this MR image. Areas of high signal represent patchy haemorrhage. The tumour extends above the sella, distorting the optic chiasma, and laterally into the right cavernous sinus.

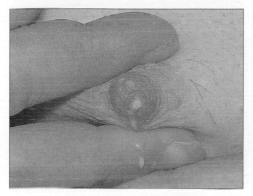

315 Galactorrhoea in a female patient with prolactinoma.

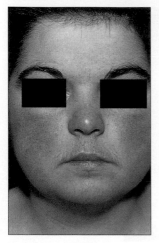

316 Cushing's syndrome. The patient has a moon face with erythema and hirsutes. Identical appearances may result from systemic costeroid therapy.

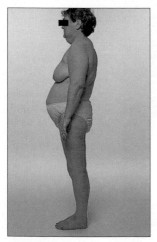

317 Cushing's syndrome results in central rather than peripheral obesity. This patient also has typical facial features and a 'buffalo hump'.

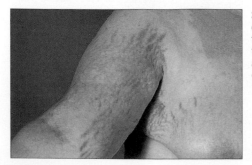

318 Cushing's syndrome. The patient has typical purple striae on the breast and arm, associated with thinning of the skin.

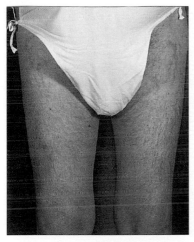

319 Proximal muscle wasting is common in Cushing's syndrome and leads to great difficult in rising from the sitting position. Note the presence of striae on both thighs.

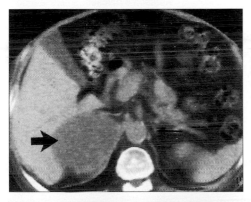

320 CT scan of a patient with an adrenal tumour causing Cushing's syndrome. The right-sided adrenal mass is marked with a thick arrow. The left adrenal gland (thin arrow) is atrophic.

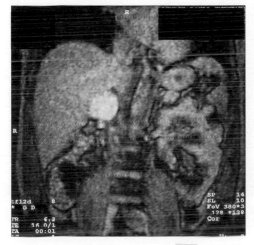

321 Phaeochromocytoma. In this coronal turboflash MR image the tumour is clearly seen as a bright circular abnormality, adjacent to the liver.

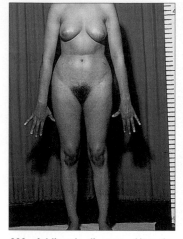

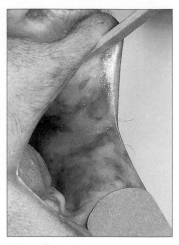

322 Addison's disease. Note the generalized increase in pigmentation, especially marked over the extensor surface of the knees.

323 Buccal pigmentation in Addison's disease. There is a general increase in mucous membrane pigmentation, and some areas of much darker pigmentation. Both features are common in Addison's disease.

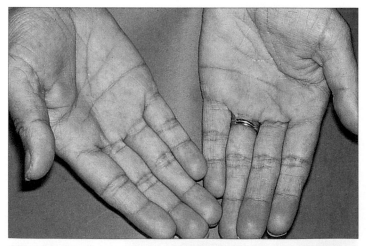

324 Addison's disease produces a marked increase in skin pigmentation in the skin creases of the hands, together with a less-marked generalized increase in pigmentation.

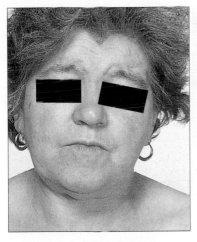

325 Hypothyroidism is not always clinically obvious. This patient shows some facial features, with a generalized pallor, puffiness and coarsening of the features, and coarse, uncontrollable hair.

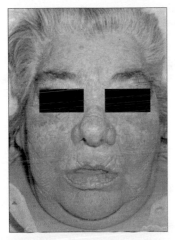

326 Gross clinical hypothyroidism produces non-pitting oedematous changes in the skin of the face, giving a characteristic clinical appearance. Note the dry, puffy facial appearance and the coarse hair.

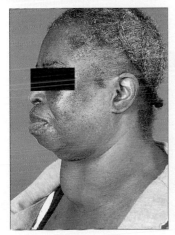

327 Endemic goitre. Large goitres like this are not unusual in areas of iodine deficiency, but they are not always associated with hypothyroidism. This African patient was euthyroid.

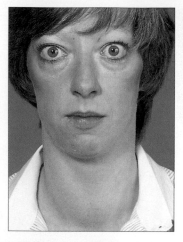

328 Hyperthyroidism – Graves' disease. This usually affects women between the ages of 20 and 40 years. This patient presented with a diffuse goitre over which a vascular bruit could be heard, and with eye signs.

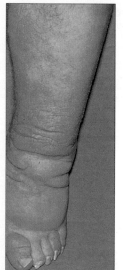

329 Pretibial myxoedema in Graves' disease. This sign may be combined with thyroid acropachy, in which there is oedema of the nail folds, producing a condition resembling clubbing.

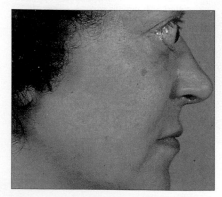

330 Exophthalmos (proptosis) in Graves' disease. This results from enlargement of the muscles, and fat within the orbit as a result of mucopolysaccharide infiltration.

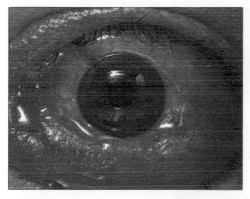

331 Severe conjunctival oedema associated with exophthalmos in a patient with Graves' disease. Tarsorrhaphy may be needed to aid lid closure and prevent damaging corneal exposure.

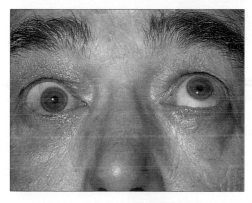

332 Ophthalmoplegia in Graves' disease is caused by swelling and infiltration of the extrinsic muscles of the eye. Here, there is impaired upward and outward gaze in the right eye. Note the lid retraction and corneal arcus.

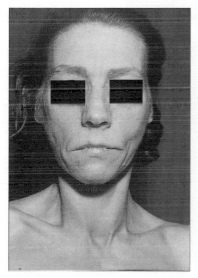

333 'Masked' hyperthyroidism. In the elderly, hyperthyroidism due to toxic multinodular goitre may be much less obvious than Graves' disease, being suggested by a combination of tachycardia, atrial fibrillation, heart failure and weight loss.

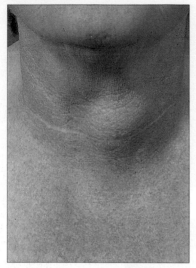

334 Toxic adenoma causing hyperthyroidism. This patient had a partial thyroidectomy 20 years previously, and a toxic nodule recurred. This was confirmed by isotope scanning.

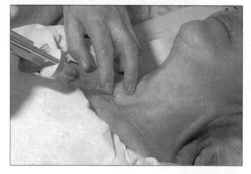

335 Fine-needle aspiration of a thyroid nodule is the investigation of choice in a patient with a solitary nodule of the thyroid, as it is very successful in obtaining cells for cytological examination.

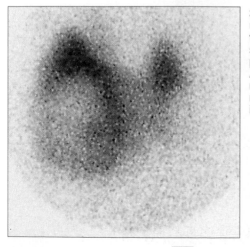

336 A large 'cold' nodule in the right lobe of the thyroid, demonstrated using ^{99m}Tc-pertechnetate scanning. A cold nodule could be malignant, and fine-needle or open biopsy is always indicated.

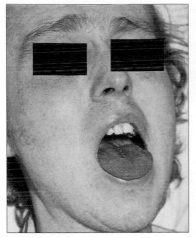

337 Diabetic ketoacidosis. There is marked dehydration. The patient was hyperventilating and confused, though not (yet) comatose. The smell of ketones on the breath allowed an instant probable diagnosis.

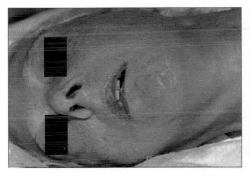

338 Hypoglycaemic coma in diabetes. Coma resulted from self-administration of excessive insulin by an alcoholic patient who did not subsequently eat any food. Hypoglycaemia is more immediately dangerous than hyperglycaemia.

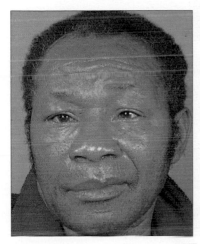

339 Acute onset mononeuritis multiplex in diabetes, affecting the right sixth and seventh facial nerves in a diabetic. The right side of the face is palsied, and the patient also had double vision on looking to the right, because a right sixth nerve palsy prevented lateral gaze in the right eye.

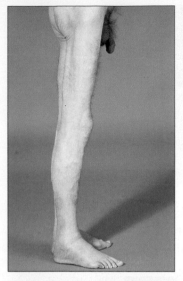

340 Diabetic amyotrophy, causing wasting of the thigh muscles. Adequate control of diabetes may lead to partial or total resolution of diabetic neuropathy.

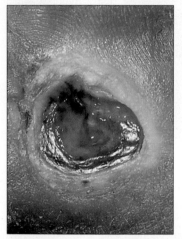

341 Painless trophic ulceration of the sole of the foot is a common presenting feature of sensory neuropathy in diabetes. Diabetic ulcers are commonly complicated by infection and gangrene.

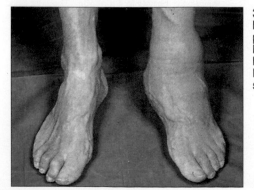

342 Charcot joint in diabetes. Sensory neuropathy has led to painless derangement of the left forefoot and ankle. Note the distortion and swelling.

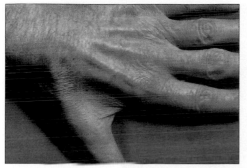

343 Ulnar mononeuro-pathy in a diabetic patient, causing wasting of the small muscles of the hand.

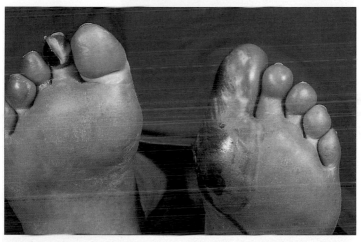

344 Gangrene of the foot is a common complication of chronic diabetes. In this patient 'wet' gangrene has developed in the hallux of the left foot, and dry gangrene in the second toe of the right foot.

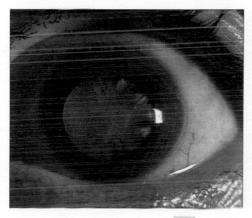

345 'Senile' cataract occurs at a younger age in diabetic patients than in the normal population. Reversible 'osmotic' cataracts may also form acutely in poorly controlled diabetics.

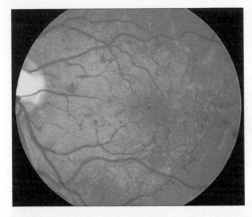

346 Background diabetic retinopathy. Note the presence of multiple microaneurysms and some small areas of haemorrhage.

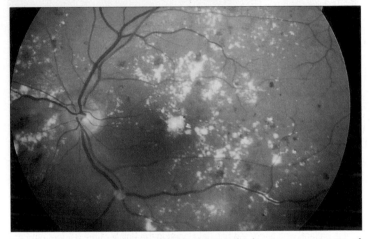

347 Macular involvement in diabetic retinopathy is a common cause of diabetic blindness. Note the presence of multiple exudates and the blurring caused by macular oedema.

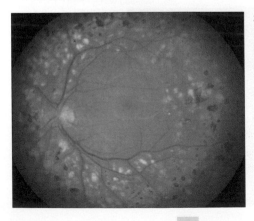

348 Photocoagulation is usually the treatment of choice for proliferative diabetic retinopathy, leaving typical scars in the peripheral retina. Many reveal the black pigmentation of the choroid beneath the destroyed retinal cells.

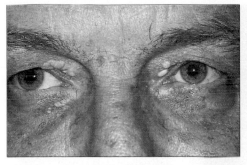

349 Hyperlipidaemia, with corneal arcus and xanthelasmata in the same patient. Even the presence of xanthelasmata alone is an indication for investigation of lipid status.

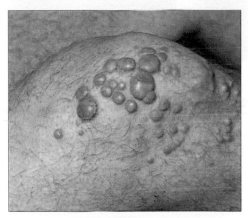

350 Tuberous xanthoma on the knee, in a patient with familial hypercholesterolaemia.

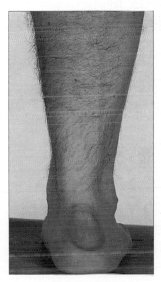

351 Tendon xanthomata are characteristically found over the tendons and extensor surfaces of joints. They are particularly common over the patellar and Achilles tendons. This patient had familial hypercholesterolaemia.

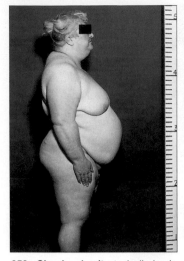

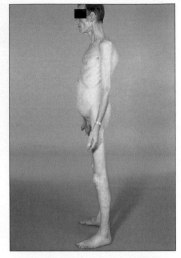

352 Simple obesity typically leads to excessive fat deposition in the upper arms, breasts, abdomen, buttocks and thighs.

353 Malnutrition has resulted in severe weight loss. Underlying malignant disease, chronic infection or malabsorption is the most likely cause, but occasionally the condition may result simply from self-neglect and inadequate food intake.

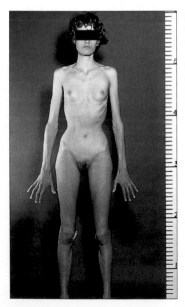

354 Anorexia nervosa in a 20-year-old woman. Note the low body weight and the preservation of breast tissue. Fine lanugo hair was present over the patient's back, and she had developed secondary amenorrhoea. Her blood pressure was 100/60 mmHg and her pukse 60/minute.

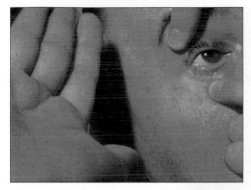

355   Carotenaemia results in an orangey pigmentation of the skin. This condition can be distinguished from jaundice by examination of the sclerae, which remain white.

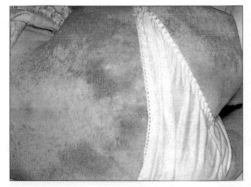

356   Zinc deficiency leads to a characteristic erythematous, hyperkeratotic skin rash. This 24-year-old woman had generalized malnutrition, associated with severe Crohn's disease.

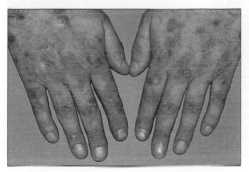

357 Porphyria cutanea tarda. Photosensitivity in this condition leads to blister formation and pigmented scarring.

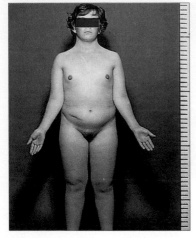

358 Turner's syndrome. Typical clinical features include retarded growth and short stature, webbed neck, absent breast development and an increased carrying angle at the elbow (cubitus valgus).

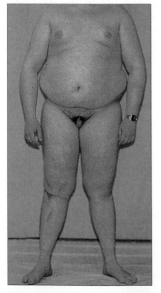

359 Klinefelter's syndrome. Patients are eunuchoid with small, firm testes, gynaecomastia and a female distribution of body hair, and they may be unusually tall.

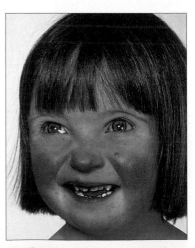

360 Down's syndrome, with prominent epicanthic folds and a small nose with a poorly developed bridge. Note also the webbed neck. This girl has Fallot's tetralogy, with a cyanosed facial flush.

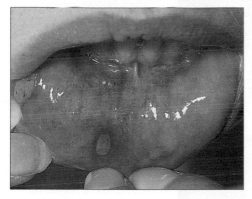

361 Aphthous ulcers commonly occur in isolation, but they may be an indication of an underlying intestinal disease, such as gluten enteropathy or inflammatory bowel disease.

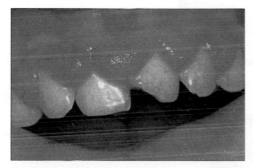

362 Hyperplastic gingivitis is a well established complication of phenytoin therapy (for epilepsy).

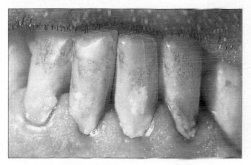

363 Lead poisoning produces a blue line at the margin of the gum and teeth. This patient presented with colicky abdominal pain.

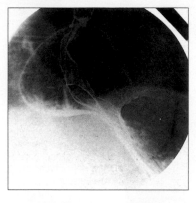

364 Rolling hiatus hernia on double-contrast barium meal. The constriction in the stomach marks the level of the diaphragm, and the gastro-oesophageal junction is still beneath it.

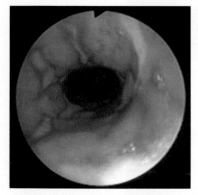

365 Peptic oesophagitis. This endoscopic view shows typical flame-like areas of shallow ulceration, coated with yellow slough. These bleed readily. Normal mucosa is present between these patches.

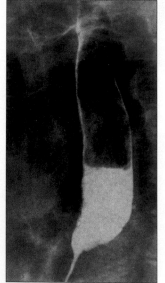

366 Benign oesophageal stricture, on barium swallow. The stricture is smooth with a tapering upper end that narrows gradually from normal oesophagus. The common cause is chronic reflux oesophagitis.

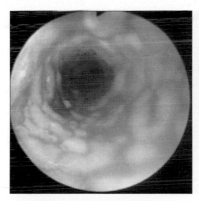

367 Oesophageal candidiasis in a patient with AIDS. The multiple small white plaques of *Candida* on the background of abnormally reddened oesophageal mucosa correspond to the radiological appearance in **8**.

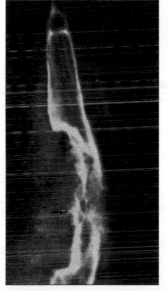

368 Oesophageal carcinoma. Note the abrupt change from normal oesophagus to the area of the tumour (cf. **366**). The barium spicules (arrows) represent areas of ulceration in the tumour.

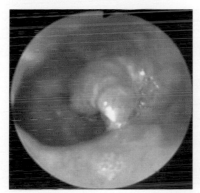

369 Carcinoma of the oesophagus seen endoscopically. The tumour is the pale sessile polypoid lesion to the right of the picture.

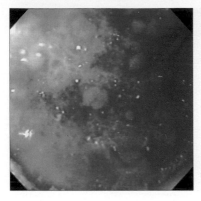

370 Acute gastritis in a patient on non-steroidal anti-inflammatory drug therapy. Multiple small erosions can be seen, and the mucosa bled when touched by the endoscope.

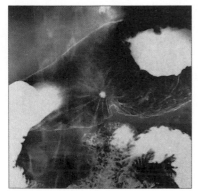

371 Benign gastric ulcer, on double-contrast barium meal. The ulcer heals by fibrosis and contraction, giving rise to the streaks of barium that radiate from the ulcer crater. Endoscopy with brush cytology or biopsy to exclude gastric carcinoma is a wise precaution, despite the benign appearance.

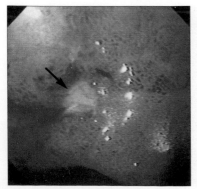

372 Benign gastric ulcer (arrow) seen on endoscopy. There is no sign of bleeding, and no evidence of malignancy, but brush cytology or biopsy is essential to exclude this.

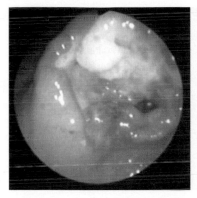

373 Carcinoma of the stomach. This ulcerated mass is situated between the incisura and the pylorus.

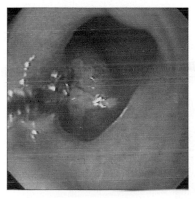

374 Endoscopic biopsy of an ulcerating mass in the stomach wall. The forceps are being advanced towards the lesion.

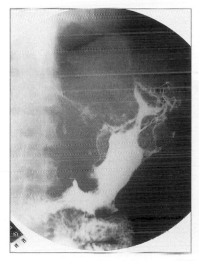

375 Carcinoma of the stomach. The barium meal demonstrates a large fungating mass in the gastric fundus. The patient presented with severe weight loss and iron-deficiency anaemia.

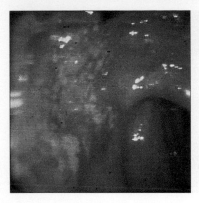

376 Duodenitis. Endoscopy shows superficial erosions of the duodenal mucosa on a background of inflammation, but no frank ulceration.

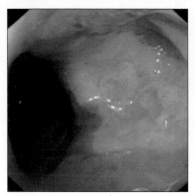

377 A large duodenal ulcer, seen via a videoendoscope.

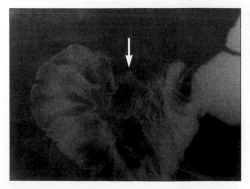

378 A small duodenal ulcer crater on double-contrast barium meal (arrow). In expert hands, this technique has a dianostic accuracy similar to that of endoscopy.

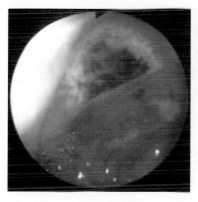

379 Haemorrhage is one of the most common complications of peptic ulceration. Adherent blood clot on a large duodenal ulcer provides evidence of recent bleeding.

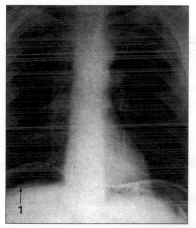

380 Pneumoperitoneum in a patient with a rigid abdomen caused by a perforated duodenal ulcer. Note the upper edge of the liver (1), and the air under both diaphragms.

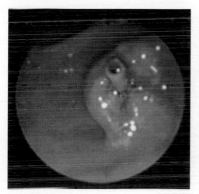

381 Carcinoma of the ampulla of Vater causing obstruction, which has been relieved by insertion of a stent. This palliative procedure can often be accomplished using a side-viewing endoscope.

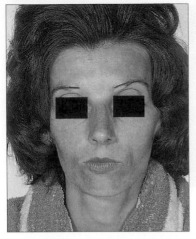

382 Coeliac disease in an adult. On presentation she weighed 40 kg (88 lb), had marked steatorrhoea and was pale and anaemic. Small bowel biopsy showed villous atrophy.

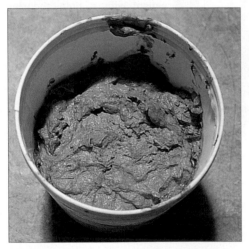

383 Typical steatorrhoea in malabsorption. The stool is pale, with the consistency of pale clay. It often floats in the lavatory and is difficult to flush away.

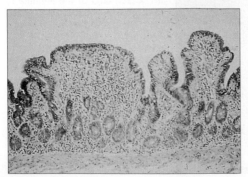

384 Jejunal biopsy from a patient with coeliac disease. The normal intestinal villi are absent, the mucosa is flattened and there is hyperplasia of the intestinal crypts. There is lymphocytic infiltration, and the surface mucosa is cuboidal rather than columnar.

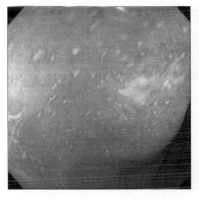

385 Crohn's proctitis. There are multiple small ulcers but the adjacent mucosa looks normal. This is a common endoscopic appearance in the rectum and colon in early Crohn's disease, although initially the ulcers may be fewer in number or even single.

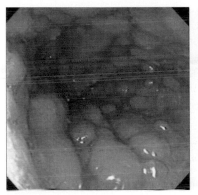

386 Crohn's disease in the colon. Multiple oedematous inflammatory polyps give a 'cobblestone' appearance to the mucosa. Similar changes may be seen in ulcerative colitis.

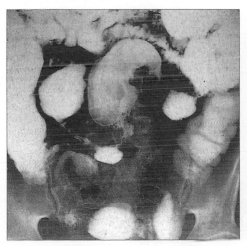

387 Crohn's disease of the small intestine revealed on barium follow-through. Four strictures of the small intestine are clearly seen, and the dilated segments of bowel appear between strictures. These 'skip lesions' are characteristic.

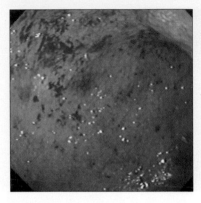

388 Ulcerative colitis. The loss of haustrations in the colon is obvious, and multiple bleeding ulcers are present. Endoscopy is hazardous in severe ulcerative colitis.

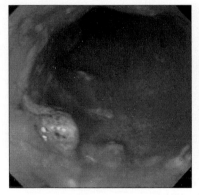

389 Inflammatory polyps ('pseudopolyps') are invariably found in the progression of ulcerative colitis. They are composed of granulomatous tissue and are highly vascular.

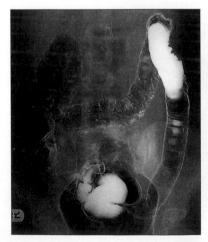

390 Ulcerative colitis. This double-contrast barium enema shows loss of the normal haustral pattern, deep penetrating ulcers, especially in the barium-filled splenic flexure, and many pseudopolyps, especially in the transverse colon.

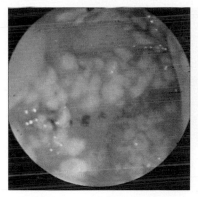

391 Pseudomembranous colitis. There are multiple yellow plaques and inflammatory changes. *Clostridium difficile* and its toxin are found in the stools.

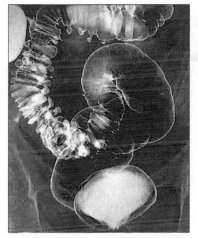

392 Diverticular disease of the colon. This barium enema shows typical changes, with multiple diverticula outlined by the double-contrast technique.

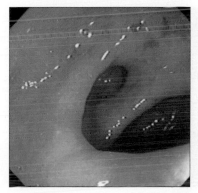

393 Severe diverticular disease viewed through the colonoscope. Wide-mouthed openings to diverticula are present.

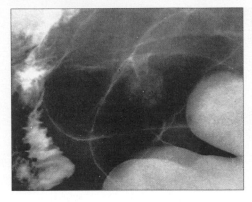

394 A single colonic polyp, beautifully revealed by double-contrast barium enema. Its pedunculated nature should mean that it can be successfully removed by snare diathermy performed through the colonoscope (see **395**).

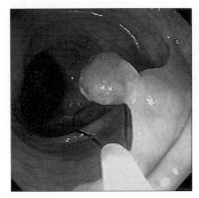

395 Colonoscopic polypectomy. A wire snare, introduced through the colonoscope, will be looped over the pedunculated colonic polyp and tightened around its stalk; diathermy will then be applied via the snare to sever the stalk without bleeding.

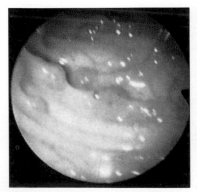

396 Familial polyposis coli. Multiple sessile polyps are seen in this colonoscopic view. There is a high risk of malignant change.

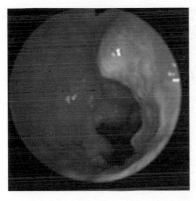

397 Colonic carcinoma seen through a colonoscope. This patient with a sessile lesion in the descending colon presented with frank bleeding.

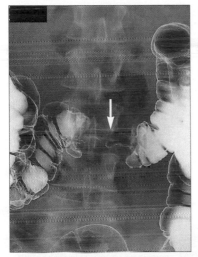

398 Colonic carcinoma in the transverse colon, revealed by double-contrast barium enema. This annular carcinoma has produced a characteristic apple-core appearance (arrow). The patient presented with chronic iron-deficiency anaemia.

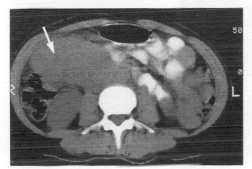

399 CT scan demonstrating a large abdominal tumour. CT-guided biopsy may permit histological diagnosis.

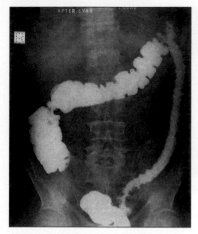

400 Colonic ischaemia. This single-contrast barium enema shows narrowing of the lumen, typical 'rose-thorn' ulcers (1) and some 'thumb-printing' (2) in the sigmoid colon, where a partial stricture has formed. The apparent stricture at the hepatic flexure disappeared on screening.

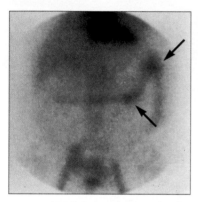

401 A bleeding site in the colon, revealed by scanning after IV administration of some of the patient's red blood cells that had been labelled with ^{99m}Tc. This 10 minute film shows two 'hot spots' in the colon (arrowed). The 'hot spot' at the splenic flexure was consistently seen in other views, and the patient was found to have a small angioma.

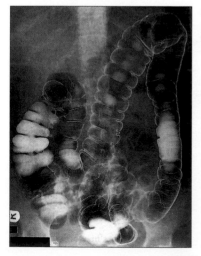

402 A normal barium enema, as seen in the irritable bowel syndrome (IBS). Colonoscopy also reveals no abnormal findings in IBS.

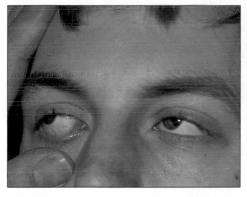

403 Acute viral hepatitis. This 19-year-old man presented with a 7-day history of malaise, nausea and vomiting and was found to be mildly jaundiced on examination.

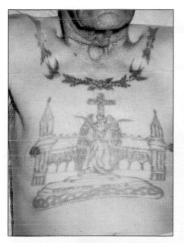

404 Tattooing is an important route of transmission for viral hepatitis and other infections including HIV. This patient developed acute hepatitis B after being tattooed and became a long-term carrier of the hepatitis B virus.

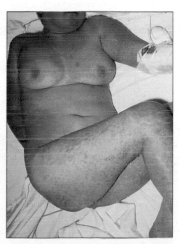

405 Drug-induced hepatitis. This patient developed severe hepatitis soon after starting phenytoin therapy. The hepatitis was accompanied by a morbilliform rash. She made a full recovery after withdrawal of phenytoin.

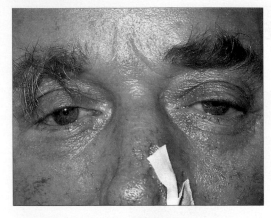

406 Acute alcoholic hepatitis. The patient presented with sudden onset jaundice. He had a history of several previous admissions after alcoholic excess.

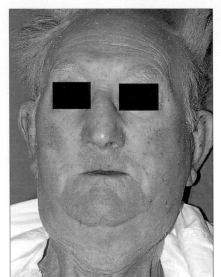

407 Parotid enlargement in association with cirrhosis is most common when alcohol is the cause of the cirrhosis. This patient also had multiple vascular spiders and early acne rosacea.

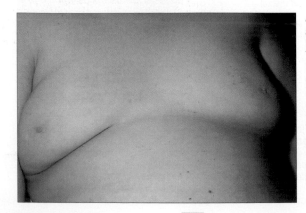

408 Chronic active hepatitis. The elevated level of conjugated bilirubin, produces a deeper yellow colour than unconjugated bilirubin. Note the associated gynaecomastia.

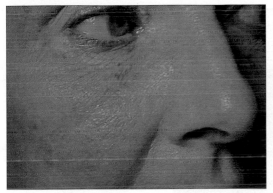

409 Primary biliary cirrhosis (PBC). The high level of conjugated bilirubin, maintained over a long period, gives a characteristic dark brown-orange pigmentation to the skin and sclerae. Note also the large xanthelasmata.

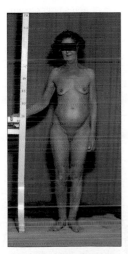

410 Primary biliary cirrhosis. This 55-year-old woman had deep jaundice, typical brown pigmentation, spider naevi, enlargement of the liver and spleen, and ascites.

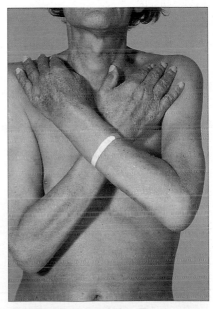

411 Haemochromatosis. The slatey-grey colour of this Caucasian patient's skin, most obvious in his hands, results from the deposition of a combination of melanin and iron. Note also the absence of body hair, associated with hypogonadism.

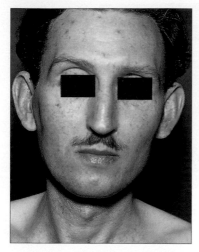

412 Spider naevi. The occurrence of a large number of spider naevi points strongly to underlying liver disease, though occasional solitary spiders may be found in normal people. This barman had alcoholic cirrhosis.

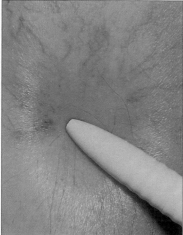

413 A spider naevus consists of a central spiral arteriole, which supplies a radiating group of small vessels. This spider naevus is of typical size, though larger and smaller examples may occur.

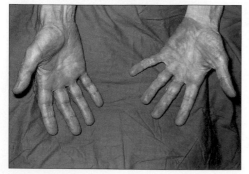

414 Palmar erythema is a common finding in chronic liver disease, but is also found in pregnancy, during oral contraceptive use, in rheumatoid arthritis, in thyrotoxicosis and as an isolated abnormality.

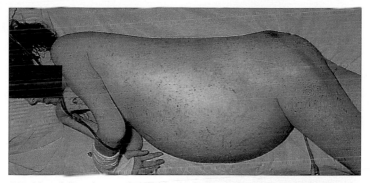

415 Liver failure in a patient with alcoholic cirrhosis. There is a gross distention of the abdomen due to severe ascites, and visible superficial dilated veins, with blood flow from the umbilicus outwards. There is also atrophy of the muscles of both upper and lower limbs. The patient was icteric, and she had fetor hepaticus. There is a large pressure sore over her left gluteal region.

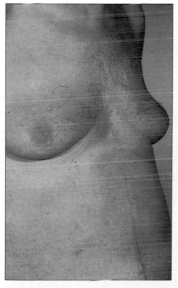

416 Gynaecomastia in a male patient. This patient had cirrhosis, and a hepatocellular carcinoma.

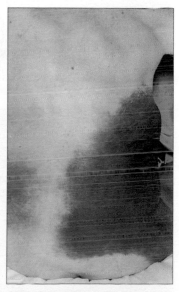

417 Spontaneous bruising in a patient with cirrhosis. Disturbance of coagulation mechanisms is a common problem in chronic liver disease.

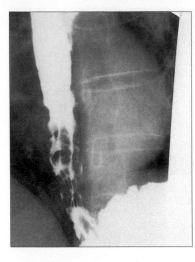

418 Oesophageal varices on barium swallow, showing the typical barium-coated filling defects. Gastric varices can also be seen, along the lesser curvature of the stomach.

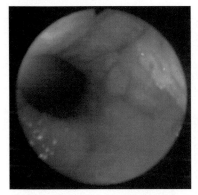

419 Varices may occur in the gastric fundus in portal hypertension. In this patient the gastric varices (to the right of the picture) are above the diaphragm in a hiatus hernia.

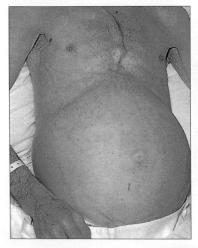

420 A peritoneovenous shunt in a patient with cirrhosis and severe ascites. The subcutaneous course of the valved shunt is clearly seen. The shunt has helped to maintain his serum albumin level, but this patient still has severe ascites.

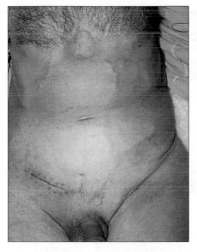

421 The Budd–Chiari syndrome (hepatic venous obstruction). Note the grossly dilated veins in the abdominal wall, in which the flow of blood was upwards. The patient was admitted with coincidental appendicitis.

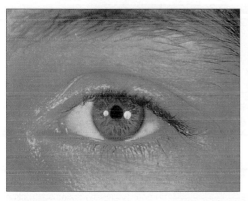

422 Wilson's disease. The impaired liver function and neurological disorder are usually accompanied by Kayser–Fleischer rings in the corneae. The rings show as a rim of brown pigment.

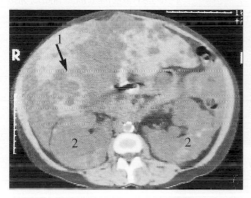

423 Polycystic liver disease, on CT scanning. The patient has massive hepatomegaly, and a typical example of the many cysts in the liver is arrowed (1). She also had bilateral polycystic kidneys (2).

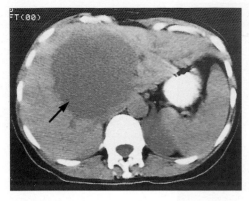

424 Primary hepato-cellular carcinoma on CT scan. The massive tumour is obvious (arrow). The liver and spleen are both enlarged. .

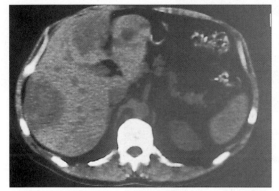

425 Multiple secondary tumour deposits of various sizes throughout the liver, shown by CT. The primary tumour was in the breast.

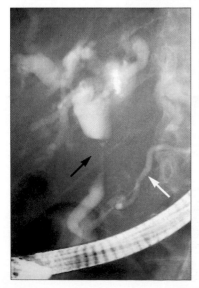

426 Cholangiocarcinoma, revealed by endoscopic retrograde cholan-giopancreatography (ERCP). The tumour is causing major obstruction of the common bile duct (black arrow). The biliary tree is grossly dilated. The pancreatic duct is also filled with contrast (white arrow).

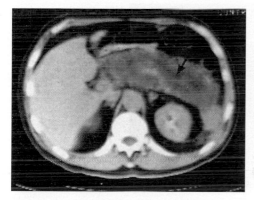

427 Acute pancreatitis. A pseudocyst in evolution can be seen in the pancreas (arrow) in this contrast-enhanced CT scan. Ultimately the cysts will coalesce to form one large pseudocyst, which may become palpable.

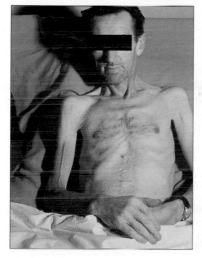

428 Chronic pancreatitis. The patient had a long history of recurrent abdominal pain. Over the past 2 years he developed steatorrhoea and weight loss, associated with pancreatic exocrine dysfunction.

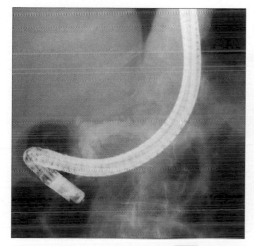

429 Endoscopic retrograde cholangiopancreatography (ERCP) in severe chronic pancreatitis. The pancreatic duct is grossly dilated and irregular. A plain film showed that some of the radio-opaque areas result from concretions within the duct system.

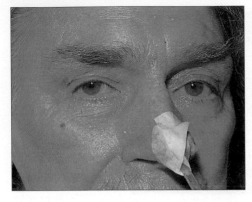

430 Carcinoma of the pancreas typically presents late in its course, as in this patient who is obviously jaundiced and has lost a considerable amount of weight, but who presented just 2 weeks before this photograph.

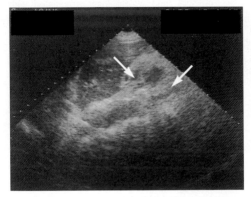

431 Pancreatic carcinoma. This ultrasound scan shows a mass in the head of the pancreas (arrows) containing several areas of decreased echogenicity, an appearance typical of carcinoma.

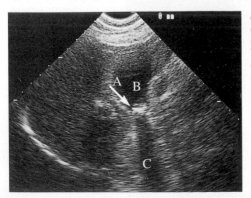

432 Ultrasound is the optimal initial investigation for gall stones. The scan shows a typical gall stone (A) in the gall bladder (B). The acoustic shadow (C) cast by the stone is typical.

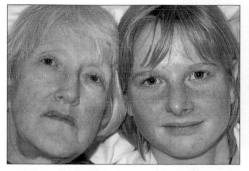

433 Clinical examination is not always a reliable guide to the haemoglobin level. The patient (on the left) had pernicious anaemia with a haemoglobin of 5.0 g/dl but she does not look exceptionally pale when compared with the normal individual on the right.

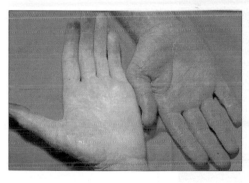

434 Pallor of the hand in anaemia is obvious in this patient, especially when compared with the physician's hand on the right.

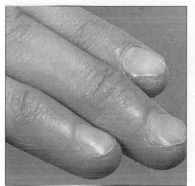

435 Pallor of the nailbeds is said to be characteristic of anaemia, but is often difficult to assess. This patient also has early koilonychia.

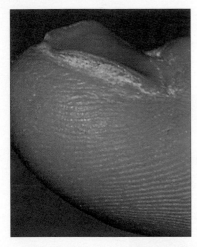

436 Koilonychia or 'spooning' of the nails is a result of a non-haemopoietic effect of iron deficiency.

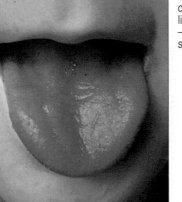

437 Iron deficiency anaemia commonly leads to pallor of the face, lips and tongue, and – when chronic – to atrophic glossitis and angular stomatitis.

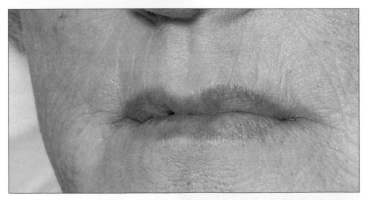

438 Angular stomatitis in a patient with iron-deficiency anaemia. Like other signs of anaemia, this is non-specific.

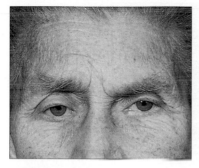

439 Pernicious anaemia often gives rise to characteristic pallor with a lemon-yellow tinge. Typically, patients with pernicious anaemia have blue eyes and (often prematurely) grey hair.

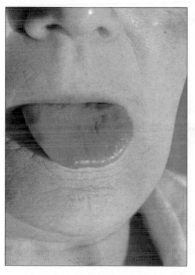

440 Pernicious anaemia. This patient has lemon-yellow skin coloration and a 'raw beef' tongue. The surface is smooth, with an absence of filiform papillae.

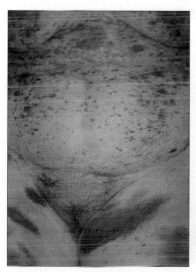

441 Aplastic anaemia. Thrombocytopenia is responsible for the widespread purpura and ecchymoses, and the patient also had a severe throat infection as a result of her low white cell count.

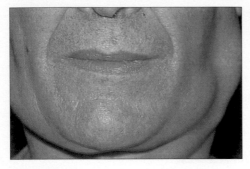

442 **Haemolytic anaemia may lead to a characteristic lemon-yellow jaundice,** as in this man who developed warm autoimmune haemolysis in association with chronic lymphocytic leukaemia. He also has cervical lymphadenopathy.

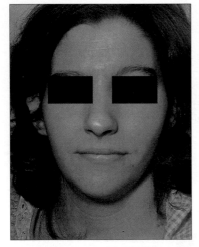

443 **Secondary haemochromatosis,** giving a characteristic skin pigmentation, may be a long-term consequence of the iron overload associated with chronic haemolytic anaemia. This 19-year-old patient had α–thalassaemia and had received multiple blood transfusions.

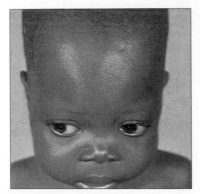

444 **Bossing of the skull, caused by hyperplasia of the bone marrow,** may occur in sickle-cell disease, thalassaemia and other severe congenital haemolytic anaemias.

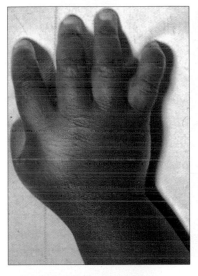

445 Severe dactylitis (inflammation of the fingers) is a common presentation of sickle-cell disease in children, and similar changes may occur in the feet.

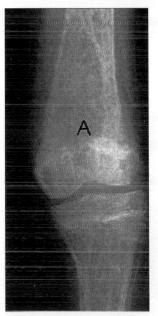

446 Thalassaemia major and sickle-cell disease may be associated with widespread marrow hyperplasia. The distal femur in this patient is expanded, giving a 'flask shaped' appearance. The bones are generally osteopenic (A), with a sparse, coarse, dense trabecular pattern.

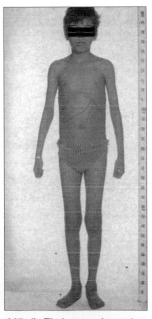

447 β–Thalassaemia major. Hepatosplenomegaly is usual, as in this young patient.

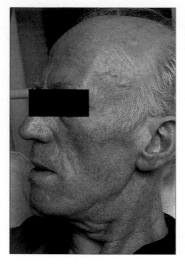

448 Primary proliferative polycythaemia (polycythaemia rubra vera). The patient has a generalized plethoric appearance, most obvious on, but not confined to, the face. Note that he also has a prominent temporal artery, which raises the possibility of temporal arteritis.

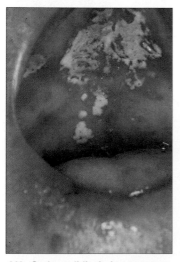

449 Oral candidiasis is a common complication of acute leukaemia. This patient also has multiple petechiae on the palate, tongue and lips and some small nodules of leukaemic infiltrate near the lower lip.

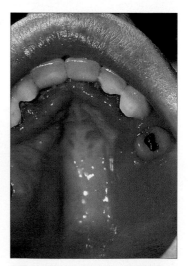

450 Infiltration of the gums is a common feature of acute leukaemia. Secondary infection often exacerbates the swelling, and bleeding is common.

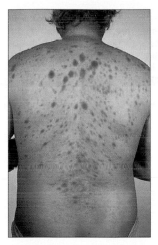

451 Extensive leukaemic infiltration of the skin may sometimes occur – most commonly in patients with acute myeloblastic leukaemia.

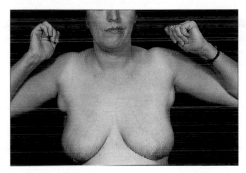

452 Chronic lymphocytic leukaemia often leads to widespread lymph node enlargement. In this patient the presenting feature was bilateral axillary lymphadenopathy.

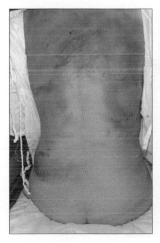

453 Excessive bruising after trauma in a patient with a myelodysplastic syndrome. This lady's bruising was excessive for the described trauma. Marrow examination showed that she had refractory anaemia with ringed sideroblasts, RAB type.

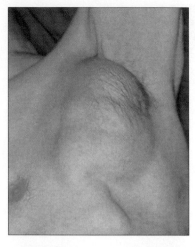

454 Gross, painless, rubbery lymph node enlargement is the common presenting feature of Hodgkin's disease. This patient's left axillary nodes were particularly prominent.

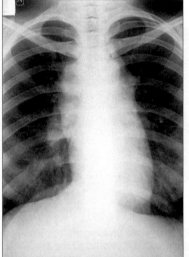

455 Chest X-ray in a patient with Hodgkin's disease, showing bilaterally enlarged mediastinal lymph nodes.

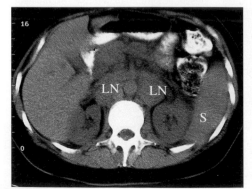

456 Hodgkin's disease. This CT scan of the abdomen shows enlargement of the spleen (S) and bilateral para-aortic lymph node enlargement (LN) at the level of the superior mesenteric artery.

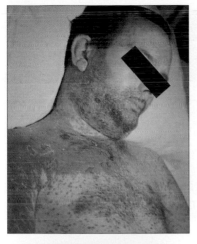

457 Widespread herpes zoster infection in a 38-year-old man with advanced Hodgkin's disease. Note that he has also developed a generalized chickenpox rash over the unaffected segments.

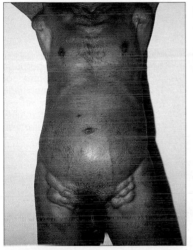

458 Non-Hodgkin's lymphoma in a patient with HIV infection. There is massive axillary and inguinal lymphadenopathy and gross hepatosplenomegaly and ascites.

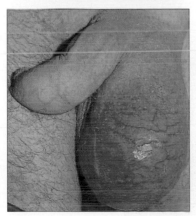

459 Lymphoma of the testis is the most common testicular neoplasm in the elderly. Patients usually present with swelling of the testis and cord up into the abdomen.

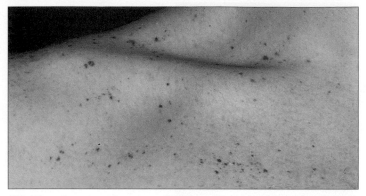

460 Thrombocytopenic purpura (TP). A number of drugs may induce TP, but the disorder is usually reversible if the drug therapy is stopped.

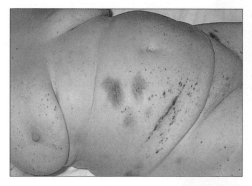

461 Diffuse purpuric rash with areas of sheet haemorrhage (ecchymosis) in a patient with thrombo-cytopenia of unknown cause.

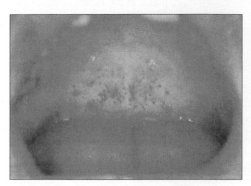

462 Petechiae on the soft palate may be a sign of thrombocyto-penic purpura. Similar transient appearances may occur harmlessly during the course of the common cold or other viral throat infections.

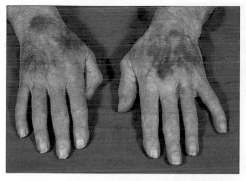

463 Senile purpura is a common and benign condition that results from impaired collagen production and capillary fragility in the elderly.

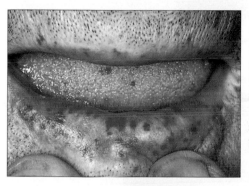

464 Hereditary haemorrhagic telangiectasia (HHT) is a condition in which occult blood loss in the gut may lead to severe iron-deficiency anaemia. The telangiectases are not always as obvious as in this patient with multiple lesions on the face, lips and tongue.

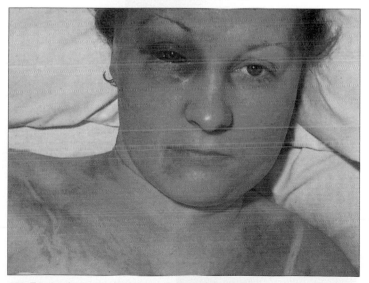

465 Traumatic asphyxia may produce severe petechiae and frank haemorrhage. This woman was crushed in a crowd, and on admission was unconscious as a result of cerebral petechiae and oedema.

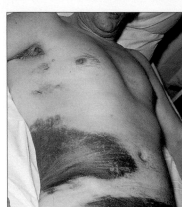

466 Massive haematomas in a patient with haemophilia. In the absence of major trauma, haematomas of this size always indicate a severe coagulation abnormality.

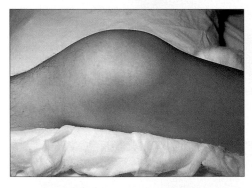

467 Acute haemarthrosis of the knee is a common complication of haemophilia. It may be confused with acute infection unless the patient's coagulation disorder is known, because the knee is hot, red, swollen and painful.

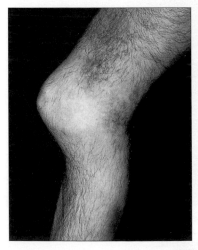

468 Genu recurvatum is a severe deformity of the knee that results from destruction of the joint by recurrent haemarthrosis. Note also the presence of acute skin haemorrhage in this haemophiliac patient.

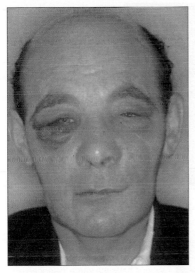

469 Spontaneous black eye in a patient on poorly controlled anti-coagulant therapy. He reported no trauma to his eye, and his INR was grossly elevated.

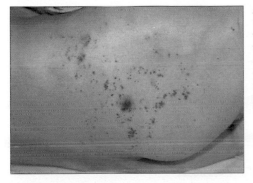

470 Disseminated intravascular coagulation (DIC) resulting from staphylococcal septicaemia. Note the characteristic skin haemorrhage ranging from small purpuric lesions to larger ecchymoses.

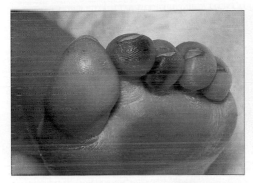

471 Peripheral gangrene can be a feature of DIC, as the balance between thrombosis and haemorrhage will vary from one part of the body to another and time to time.

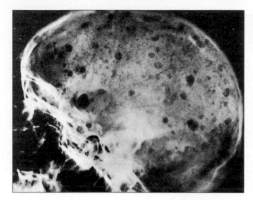

472 Myeloma lesions in bones show up as characteristic 'punched out' lesions without surrounding sclerosis. Secondary deposits from other tumours may occasionally give a similar appearance.

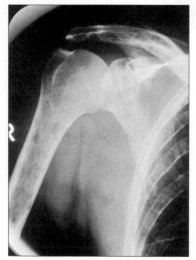

473 Myeloma in the humerus, scapula, clavicle and ribs. The lesions have the same 'punched out' appearance as those seen in the skull. Pathological fractures may occur, and hypercalcaemia is common.

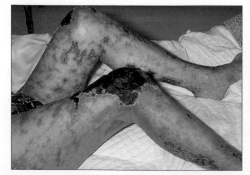

474 Skin infarction in cryoglobulinaemia. There is a reticulated pattern to the skin due to leakage of red cells from damaged skin capillaries. Necrosis and ulceration has occurred in peripheral sites due to vessel blockage.

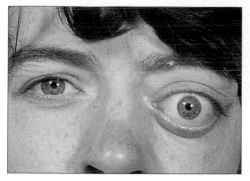

475 Unilateral proptosis resulted from a meningioma on the sheath of the optic nerve in this patient. Exophthalmos in Graves' disease, is usually bilateral.

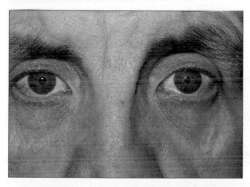

476 Argyll Robertson pupils are a feature of tertiary neurosyphilis and occasionally, of diabetes. They are small, irregular and unresponsive to light, but they react normally on accommodation.

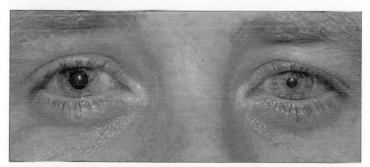

477 Holmes–Adie pupil in the right eye of a young woman. The affected pupil is 'tonic', responding slowly to light and accommodation, but on rapid testing will appear unresponsive.

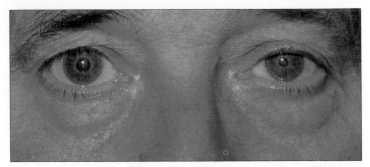

478 Horner's syndrome showing ptosis of the left eye, associated with constriction of the pupil (miosis). This patient had syringomyelia.

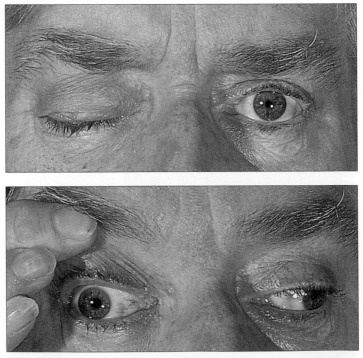

479 & 480 Third nerve palsy with complete right ptosis. In the resting position, the right eye was rotated laterally and downwards (**479**). The palsy was the result of compression of the third cranial nerve by an aneurysm of the posterior communicating artery. When the patient looks to the left the right eye has rotated to the midposition (**480**), demonstrating that the trochlear (fourth) nerve is intact.

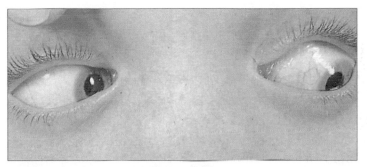

481 Right fourth nerve palsy demonstrated on looking down and to the left. This movement is impaired in the right eye. The patient presented with diplopia.

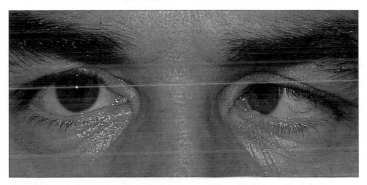

482 Right sixth nerve palsy. The right eye fails to abduct on lateral gaze.

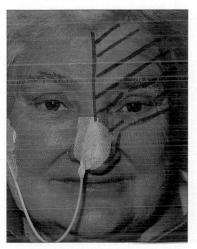

483 Trigeminal nerve palsy, affecting the ophthalmic division of the nerve. The distribution of sensory impairment is marked.

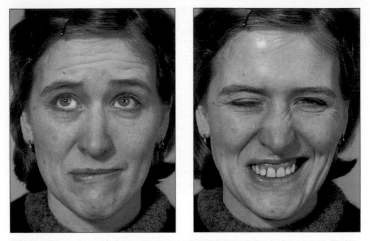

484 & 485 Lower motor neurone palsy of the right facial nerve (Bell's palsy). This patient is unable to wrinkle her brow fully on the affected side, the right corner of her mouth droops and there is a prominent right nasolabial fold (**484**). When the patient is asked to close her eyes and show her teeth (**485**), the difference between the unaffected left side and the affected right side becomes more obvious.

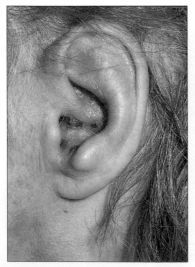

486 The Ramsay Hunt syndrome presents with facial palsy identical to Bell's palsy, and with herpetic vesicles in the external auditory meatus.

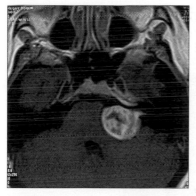

487 Acoustic neuroma. A large tumour at the left cerebellopontine angle, demonstrated by gadolinium enhancement on axial MRI scan.

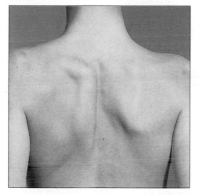

488 Accessory nerve palsy. The right trapezius does not contract when the patient shrugs his shoulders, and examination also revealed paralysis of the right sternomastoid muscle.

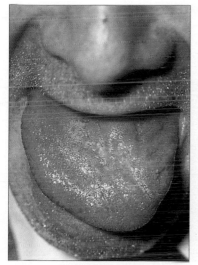

489 Left hypoglossal nerve palsy. This patient presented with deviation of the tongue to the affected side when it was pushed out, associated with fasciculation and fissuring caused by wasting.

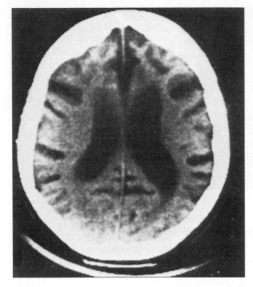

490 CT scan in Alzheimer's disease. Note the marked dilatation of the sulci and fissures, especially frontally, the poor distinction between grey matter and white matter, the ventricular enlargement and the general reduction in brain size.

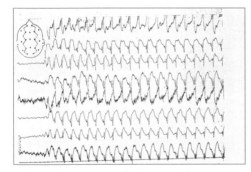

491 EEG in a patient with generalized seizures. This shows the typical spike and wave discharge of epilepsy. If the EEG is taken during an attack, this appearance may be diagnostic of epilepsy.

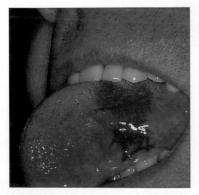

492 The bitten tongue as a sign of epilepsy. Damage to the tongue is a common complication of generalized seizures.

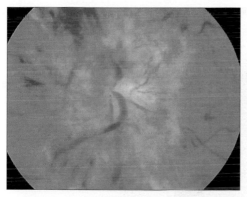

493 Chronic papilloedema in the right eye of a middle-aged woman with benign intracranial hypertension. The disc margins are completely blurred, and there are widespread haemorrhages and ischaemic areas in the retina.

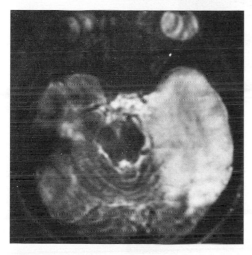

494 Herpes simplex encephalitis. This MRI view shows abnormally increased signal in the left temporal lobe (right of picture).

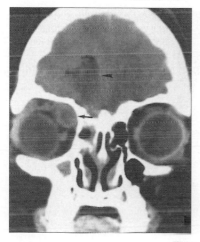

495 Cerebral abscess secondary to ethmoid sinusitis. This coronal CT scan demonstrates the frontal abscess (arrowhead) and also an abscess in the orbit (arrow)

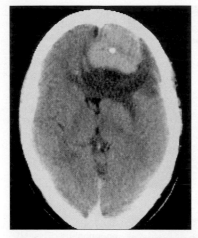

496 Contrast enhanced CT scan showing a left frontal meningioma, with the classic appearance of a densely enhancing, sharply marginated tumour, tightly against the dura.

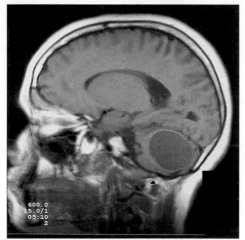

497 A large cerebellar cyst in MRI sagittal view. MRI is of particular value in demonstrating lesions in the posterior fossa.

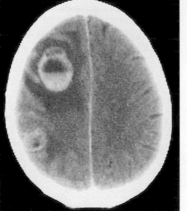

498 Multiple cerebral metastases in a patient with carcinoma of the bronchus, demonstrated on CT scan. 'Cuts' at other levels in the brain demonstrated further lesions.

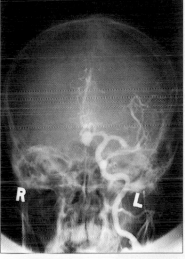

499 Subarachnoid haemorrhage from an anterior communicating artery aneurysm. This uncontrasted CT scan shows areas of increased density representing blood in the interhemispheric fissure (arrows), in the septum pellucidum (arrowheads), the sylvian fissures and the perimesencephalic cistern.

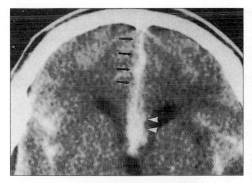

500 Berry aneurysm on the anterior communicating artery. The patient presented with a subarachnoid haemorrhage.

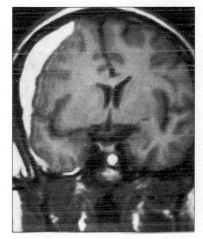

501 Right subdural haemorrhage revealed by MRI. The high intensity (white) haemorrhage has dissected under the temporal lobe, and the midline has been displaced to the left.

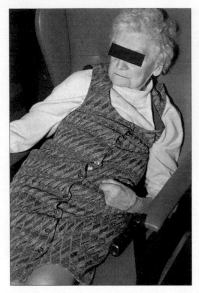

502 Loss of postural stability is common after stroke. The patient is unable to sit upright and tends to fall sideways.

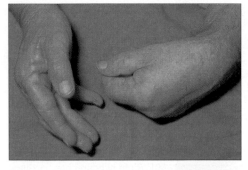

503 Disuse oedema is a common long-term complication of stroke. In this patient, the left hand remains swollen months after the onset of a dense hemiplegia.

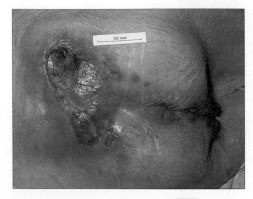

504 Severe sacral pressure sore – one of the serious but preventable complications of immobility following stroke. Note also the presence of a urinary catheter, commonly associated with recurrent urinary infections.

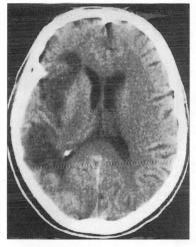

505 Extensive right-sided cerebral infarction (left side of picture) demonstrated by unenhanced CT scan, performed 4 days after the onset of stroke.

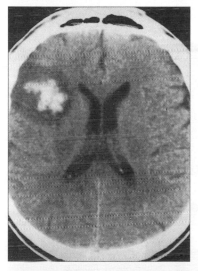

506 Haemorrhagic cerebral infarction demonstrated in the right hemisphere by unenhanced CT scan on day 1. Note the high-density haemorrhage within the low density of the oedematous, infarcted region.

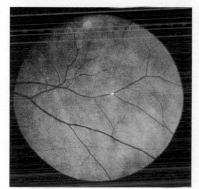

507 Retinal embolus in a patient with transient ischaemic attacks. Emboli may sometimes be seen in the retina in patients who have symptoms suggesting a TIA.

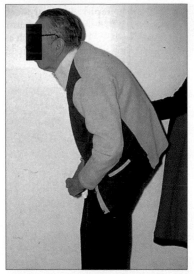

508 Parkinson's disease – typical posture and gait. Note the stoop and the typical flexion of the arms.

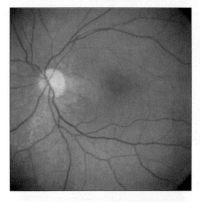

509 Retrobulbar neuritis is a common initial presentation of multiple sclerosis. The disc may develop papillitis with blurred margins and occasional haemorrhages and later may develop the pallor of optic atrophy.

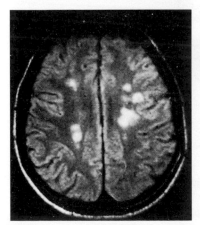

510 Multiple sclerosis. This MRI picture shows multiple 'high signal' lesions in the white matter of both hemispheres. These represent multiple areas of demyelination.

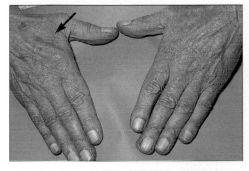

511 Motor neurone disease presents with progressive muscular atrophy, fasciculation and wasting of the muscles between the thumb and index finger on the dorsal (arrow) and palmar surfaces.

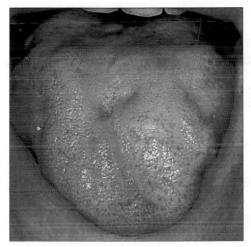

512 Motor neurone disease. This patient had progressive bulbar palsy. An early feature was fasciculation of the tongue, followed by progressive wasting, with furrowing of the surface.

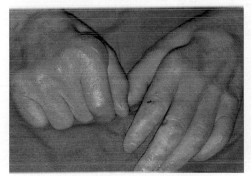

513 Syringomyelia. The patient has severe wasting of the small muscles of both hands. He has also sustained a painless burn at the base of the right index finger.

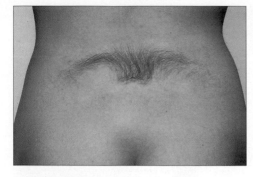

514 Occult spina bifida may be suggested by the presence of a tuft of hair over the base of the spine. This is usually harmless anomaly, but may be associated with diastematomyelia.

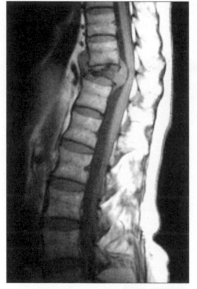

515 Compression of the spinal cord leading to paraplegia. The MRI shows complete collapse of a vertebra with consequent cord compression, as a result of a secondary deposit.

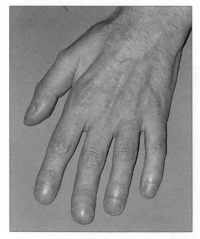

516 Wasting of the hand as a consequence of ulnar neuropathy. Note the marked wasting of the interosseous muscles, especially the first dorsal interosseous.

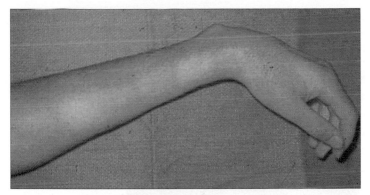

517 Radial nerve palsy. The patient is unable to extend the wrist and the metacarpophalangeal joints of the fingers or thumb – he has 'wrist drop'.

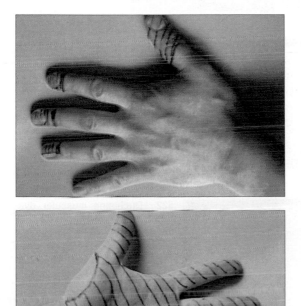

518, 519 Carpal tunnel syndrome. The common areas of sensory impairment are marked in this patient. Note that they usually extend round the fingertips on to the nail area in the affected fingers and even further over the extensor surface on the thumb. Wasting of the thenar eminence is also seen.

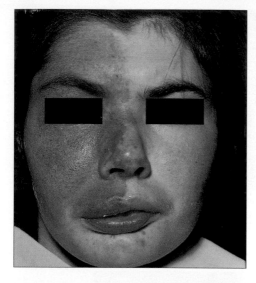

520 Sturge–Weber syndrome. This patient has a classic diffuse capillary haemangioma in the distribution of the ophthalmic, nasociliary and maxillary branches of the trigeminal nerve.

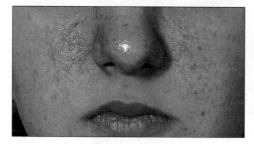

521 Adenoma sebaceum of the face – a marker of tuberous sclerosis (epiloia). The lesions are angiofibromas, and these are associated with mental retardation, epilepsy and other skin changes.

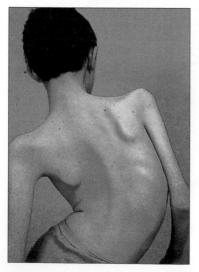

522 Duchenne muscular dystrophy. This 15-year-old boy has severe scoliosis and an equinovarus deformity of the feet.

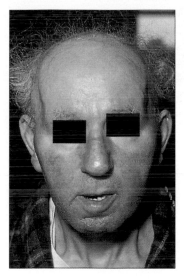

523 Myotonic dystrophy in a 50-year-old man. His appearance is typical, with facial weakness, atrophy of the temporal muscles and sternomastoids and frontal baldness.

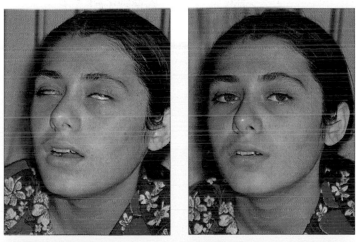

524 & 525 Myasthenia gravis. Facial weakness is provoked by repeated facial movements (**524**). Edrophonium chloride (Tensilon), a short-acting anticholinesterase, is then injected intravenously – initially 2 mg as a test dose, followed after 1 minute by a further 8 mg if there are no adverse effects. In myasthenia gravis the facial weakness is rapidly relieved by this test (**525**).

INDEX